Secrets of
AYURVEDIC MASSAGE

Atreya

LOTUS PRESS

Dedication

*Special thanks to Vamadeva Shastri, without your
support and help in understanding Ayurveda, Yoga and
the Vedic sciences this book would not be possible.
You are a gift to all students of the ancient Vedic knowledge.*

And to my beloved Girija, everpure and stainless.

COPYRIGHT © 2000 By ATREYA

COVER & PAGE DESIGN/LAYOUT: Paul Bond, Art & Soul Design

PHOTOGRAPHY: Luc Baby

First Edition, 2000

Printed in the United States of America

Library of Congress Cataloging-in-Publication-Data
Ayurvedic Massage, Self-Healing and Self-Realization
includes bibliographical references.
ISBN 0-914955-49-7   99-75332
                                                                   CIP

Published by:
Lotus Press, P.O. Box 325, Twin Lakes, Wisconsin 53181
web: www.lotuspress.com
e-mail: lotuspress@lotuspress.com
800-824-6396

Table of Contents

Introduction

*"Things that are inconceivable should not be subject to
canons of logic; and this world is one such, for the mind
cannot conceive of the very mode of its creation"*
—Pancadasi, VI-150

Touch is a form of communication. As such,
any form of touch communicates a message.
This book explains how to transmit a powerful therapeutic message in massage. This is possible because the Ayurvedic system
of health care provides the most comprehensive therapeutic structure for massage in the world.

The essence of understanding the Ayurvedic system is to understand *prana*. There is nothing more subtle in the body than
prana. Even a subtle mental process like thinking can be grasped,
reasoned with or utilized. Not so with *prana*. It is untouchable
and unknowable. It empowers the body/mind and is closely linked
with the soul. Prana manifests as the three humors in Ayurveda.

Without a good understanding of Prana and its fivefold functions in the body, Ayurvedic massage cannot be understood as a
therapeutic science. As with many of the methods coming from
the Indian Vedic tradition the presentation of massage from the
Ayurvedic system is usually missing the subtle aspects that make
it a true healing therapy. These secrets set Ayurvedic massage
apart from other methods of bodywork along with its use of medicinal plants and oils. The lack of the subtle anatomy in the
system's presentation is indeed a calamity. The purpose of this
book is to clearly present the secrets behind the Ayurvedic methodology of massage and to present it as a true healing technique.

This book is also intended to give the lay person an idea of
what Ayurvedic massage is so that consumer knowledge will increase the quality of the product. Currently there are numerous

people claiming to offer 'Ayurvedic Massage' without proper knowledge of the system. This book is for these people as well - to help you best utilize the system for your work as a therapist.

This book will introduce massage techniques and offer 'hands on' practical information. However, the focus is to clearly present the subtle anatomy and medicinal techniques that make Ayurveda such a comprehensive system of understanding the body/ mind/ soul complex. The correct use of the external application of oils and herbs will also be explained in a manner suitable for Westerners. The secrets of working with the subtle energy of the body - *prana or Vayu* - will be the emphasis. In fact, the actual purpose of Ayurvedic massage is to harmonize the *Vata Dosha* or the humor that controls movement and that is the primary cause of disease.

The Place of Massage in Ayurveda

First we must understand the role of massage therapy in the Ayurvedic system. To effectively understand this we must know something of the system as a whole. It is not the purpose of this book to introduce Ayurveda as a health care system, I have covered this material in *Practical Ayurveda*.[1] Refer to the bibliography if you wish to have an introductory book on the Ayurvedic system as a whole.

Ayurvedic therapies can be divided into two distinct branches: strengthening and reducing, or *Brimhana* and *Langhana*. Strengthening therapies are relatively simple and are designed to increase the strength of the patient. Reduction therapies are reducing in nature and are more complex. Reduction therapy is usually given before strengthening therapies to clean and prepare the system for regeneration and rejuvenation. Ayurvedic massage can be used in both ways - either to strengthen the system or to help clean and reduce excess in the system.

Many people think that Ayurvedic massage is confined to lifestyle therapies or to the *Pancha Karma* therapies. Massage has a greater use than these two areas, yet massage is extremely important in lifestyle treatments and in preparing for Pancha Karma. Lifestyle therapies are those things that you do every day. What you do daily constitutes your overall health in time as it is the continuos repetition of an action that gives it power. In the context of daily habits massage is used to contain *Vata*, the

Secrets of Ayurvedic Massage

humor of wind/air, or movement.

Pancha Karma (lit. five actions) is a combination of five different reducing therapies designed to eliminate excess of the three humors. In order for these therapies to work the excess of the humors must be brought to their primary sites in the digestive tract. This is accomplished through two primary means - Oleation (the use of oil) and Sweat Therapy. The application of oil to the exterior of the body prepares it to receive the five reducing therapies of Pancha Karma. It is the oil in this therapy that is important, not the technique of massage. This system is complex and must be done with a qualified doctor of Ayurveda. Dr. Sunil Joshi explains this system completely and clearly in his book on Pancha Karma.[2] The result of Pancha Karma is the pacification of the three humors, again primarily Vata. This results in health.

Following any form of reducing therapy strengthening therapy must be given to build back, or to maintain the strength of, the patient. Pancha Karma is often seen as a 'quick fix' to Westerners which will allow them to return to a poor lifestyle after a week or two of treatment. This is so far from the truth that it is dangerous. Reducing therapy prepares your body for medicine in the form of food, herbs or ways of living. If you ingest toxic substances or keep toxic thoughts and emotions they now have a direct path to the deeper layers of the body - the site of serious diseases. Pancha Karma is a beautiful method if done correctly and if administered in the proper amount of time, i.e., three to six weeks. However, it is only marketing if a center or person is advertising a four to seven day cure using Pancha Karma. This kind of marketing can have severe effects on your health in the long term.

For the reasons above I prefer to use slow reducing therapies - such as herbs that detoxify and reduce - that do not interfere with a Western lifestyle (typically stressed out with no time for the healing process). Massage plays an important part in this approach as it does in preparing for Pancha Karma. In this book several different methods of using massage will be explained in the correct context to the Ayurvedic system as applied for the average Western person.

Purpose of Massage

While this may seem obvious, it is not. What is the purpose of giving a massage? Do you wish to relax? To release tension? To strengthen the body? To help liberate toxins? To nourish the muscle and fat tissues? To maintain the three humors? To balance one of the humors? Are you using massage as part of a greater reducing therapy? Are you using massage as part of a strengthening program? To open and release deep connective tissue? To release trapped emotions and feelings?

For any of the above reasons the constitution, or *Prakruti*, of the person must be determined, then the present state, or *Vakruti*, of the person must be determined. The purpose of giving a massage must then be defined according to a comparison of Prakruti and Vakruti, i.e., the natal constitution versus the present constitution. With this information an Ayurvedic therapy can be determined. Without understanding the therapeutic purpose - the present condition of the patient and the unique nature of the person to be treated - you are not practicing Ayurveda.

There are four primary divisions or purposes for giving a massage in Ayurveda:

- to eliminate excess
- to purify
- to strengthen or rejuvenate
- to maintain the strength

The first two fall under reducing therapies and the last two fall under strengthening therapies. The elimination of toxins and excess in the body is useful in weight management, obesity, malefactions of the digestive system, management of the *Pitta* and *Kapha* humors and general excesses in the body. This is primarily used for Kapha management and treatment, and secondarily Pitta management and treatment. Understand that as Vata provides the principle of movement in the body it is always involved with the elimination of anything as it controls elimination from the body.

Elimination works to drive out excess from the seven tissue levels of the body so that they can be taken out through purification methods. Oleation therapies are used to penetrate the tissues and liberate toxins as well as drive the humors back to their home in the intestinal tract. Oleation therapies include the internal use of oil, i.e., the drinking of oil. These methods are accom-

Secrets of Ayurvedic Massage

panied by sweat therapy. In other words deep medicated oil massages that are designed to purify the system must be used with sweat boxes or dry saunas to work effectively. This is actually a preparation for the Pancha Karma therapies. However, you can use them in certain cases very effectively without doing Pancha Karma.

Purification relates primarily to the Pancha Karma methods of removing the excess of the three humors from the body. It differs from elimination in that it essentially uses strong methods to clear the digestive system, although other methods exist. These methods work primarily on Vata and secondarily on Pitta and Kapha. Purification can also be considered the strongest form of therapy and not all persons are able to receive it. Massage does play a role in this form of therapy, but is used more before and after as preparation and post care.

Strengthening or rejuvenation therapies fall under the fortification therapies and, as mentioned earlier, are given after reducing therapies to strengthen the patient. Reducing therapies do just that - reduce. They not only reduce excesses in the body, they also reduce the overall strength and vitality. Thus, rejuvenating therapies must be given to build back the vitality of the person. This is an important part of post Pancha Karma therapies. Often strengthening therapies are given at the same time as reducing therapies if the patient doesn't have sufficient overall strength to do reducing methods alone. It is important that the therapist be able to determine the capacity of the patient before beginning any therapy. Rejuvenation therapies are also used on older people to increase their stamina and resistance to disease. These therapies work on all the humors. Light medicated oil massage is very strengthening.

Maintenance therapies fall under lifestyle treatments and are what we do daily or weekly to keep our health. In Ayurveda this is defined as keeping the three humors in balance. This method is mostly used to control Vata - which is the main cause of disease in the body. Light oil massages with herbs according to your constitution are used on a regular basis. Oil is the best substance to control Vata as it is exactly opposite to Vata in nature. Usually, Vata becomes disturbed and moves from its home and disturbs or aggravates the other two humors. Hence, maintenance of Vata is the best preventative method of illness.

With the above information in mind it is important to realize that for massage to really be considered a method of healing someone there are a number of factors to understand. Massage can be used to relax a friend or family member, to help ease tension, etc. However, this should not be confused with the actual therapy of Ayurvedic massage which, in a medical application, is more advanced than Western massage. Western massage is strong in techniques and is very sophisticated in this respect. Nevertheless, its actual medical effectiveness is far less than massage used in Ayurveda. This is primarily because massage has always been in the Ayurvedic medical system and not outside of it or ignored, as it has been in the West.

The skin is an important organ of assimilation and you should not put something on your skin that you would not put in your mouth. Ayurveda uses this knowledge from a therapeutic perspective to increase the effectiveness of its other therapies. The beauty of the Ayurvedic system is that it is not limited to the physical body, but views the inter-relatedness of nature in its totality.

The Subtle Anatomy in Massage

Certainly one of the most interesting aspects of massage in Ayurveda is that of the subtle anatomy. As Ayurveda, *Yoga* and *Jyotish* (I mean the whole Yogic tradition here of which the *asanas,* postures, of Hatha Yoga are but a very small part) are all interrelated sciences - each contributes to the other. Jyotish, the Science of Light, brings in the understanding of time and the correct timings for an activity. Ayurveda, the Science of Life, brings the knowledge of how to live in harmony with nature and to live without disease. Yoga, the Science of Union, gives the methodology to unite with the cosmic soul and along with that a complete understanding of the subtle universe.

I have a successful friend and client in Switzerland who has been practicing yoga asanas for years. Several years ago he hosted an introductory workshop on Ayurveda that I taught. He became very enthusiastic about Ayurveda and follows a rigid application of the lifestyle appropriate for his constitution. Each time I see him he asks me if I am doing yoga. By this he means if I do asanas every day, something I am relaxed about. I tried several times, without success, to explain to him that yoga asanas are not Yoga. This is somewhat like taking a few Ayurvedic herbs and saying that you are practicing Ayurveda. Yoga is a vast science that is not possible to 'practice'. Yoga is a way of being in yourself that recognizes a divine quality inherent in all living creatures. Through this recognition you strive to 'join' or become in union with this divineness. People who understand Yoga say they know nothing. People who do asanas say they understand yoga.

It is from the Yogic tradition that Ayurveda has taken the subtle anatomy, or rather, they developed side by side. Ayurveda has developed the science of the *marmas*, vital points in the body, much greater than Yoga. And Yoga has developed the understanding of the *nadis*, channels of vital force or prana, to a greater extent. In Ayurvedic massage we use both the nadis, marmas and the *chakras*.

By using the subtle anatomy of Ayurveda we can greatly increase our effectiveness as therapists. The root of this knowledge lies in prana. It is the Cosmic Prana that divides three fold into the *tridosha*, or three humors, Vata, Pitta and Kapha. These three humors control the five states of matter which creates manifest forms. Prana further divides five fold as the five Vayus, or vital airs, in the human body. These five forces control and animate the body. Nothing can function without them. Prana is synonymous with life, with soul.

Hence, we come full circle back to this unseen force that brings us health or disease. Health is brought through the right use of, or knowledge of prana in foods, herbs, water and life itself. Disease is brought through the wrong use of prana or through ignorance. The real function of this book is to eliminate this ignorance that is the prime cause of unhappiness and illness in the world.

---

[1] Atreya, *Practical Ayurveda: Secrets of Physical, Sexual & Spiritual Health*, York Beach, Me; Samuel Weiser, Inc. 1998

[2] Joshi, Dr. Sunil V., *Ayurveda and Panchakarma*, Twin Lakes, WI; Lotus Press, 1996

1 Prakruti: The Individual Nature

"Prakruti (primordial substance) is that in which there is the reflection of Brahman, that is, pure consciousness and bliss, and is composed of sattva, rajas and tamas."
—Pancadasi, I-15

The fundamental approach of Ayurveda is individualistic. Ayurveda does not treat statistics, averages or generalized groups of people. Ayurveda treats *individuals*! Ayurvedic massage places primary importance on the Prakruti (nature or constitution) of the person receiving the massage. Understanding the prakruti of a person is far more important than being an expert of techniques from the Ayurvedic standpoint. Hence, systems of massage that purport to be 'Ayurvedic' and do not teach simple methods to determine constitution are not in fact using Ayurveda.

The purpose of understanding the different constitutional types in massage is all important. If this information alone is absorbed and utilized it will change completely your present massage approach.

While it is understood that massage cannot be taught from a book, the primary, fundamental essence can be given. Understanding prakruti is the fundamental step in using Ayurvedic massage as a healing therapy.

According to the seers who developed the Ayurvedic system there are three fundamental forces that govern the manifest universe. These three forces are different forms of *Prana*. For an in-depth look at this and the role of prana in Ayurveda generally refer to *'Practical Ayurveda'*.[1] The names of these forces are metaphoric in Sanskrit and so the English translations of them should also be taken as metaphoric - indicating an unseen force, but who's action is observable. The three forces are given as Vata (wind), Pitta (bile), and Kapha (phlegm). We can loosely translate them as air, fire and water.

Rather than spend pages describing the three forces (Sanskrit - doshas, or tridosha for the three together) I will give a brief description and refer you to 'Prakruti: Your Ayurvedic Constitution' by Dr. Robert Svoboda.[2] Dr. Svoboda's book is the classic in the West for giving a profound explanation of the three doshas. The ancient Greeks took the tridosha theory from ancient India and developed their own theory of the four humors. According to the Greeks the four humors could determine a persons physical and mental qualities. Thus, the concept of the doshas have been in Western culture and thought for well over 2000 years. Hence, we need not look at the tridoshic theory as foreign to our civilization.

The three humors exist in every person. The mix of the three is what determines the individuality of people. There are seven types traditionally given. However, many people are now classifying these into ten types to be more precise in the treatment process. Within these ten types there are yet another three qualitative types that help further to determine the nature of a person. These three qualities are called *Gunas* in Sanskrit.

According to Vedic thought (of which yoga and Ayurveda are derived from) the three gunas, or qualities, are what determine the psychology of the person. This, as we know, greatly effects the physical functions of the body. So of the ten different constitutional types we can now further divide them into another three possibilities, or thirty main constitutional types. Within these thirty possible types there are infinite possibilities. The three gunas are: Sattva, Rajas, Tamas, or harmony, action, and inactivity.

Any kind of bodywork is known to release suppressed, repressed, latent, and unconscious emotions in the tissues. By understanding the three gunas the practitioner can have a deeper insight into the quality and type of stored emotion. While it is usually not the direct focus of Ayurvedic massage to release stored emotions, any practitioner will be aware that it happens anyway and is often the prime cause of regaining health. I will endeavor to explain how this can be viewed from the Ayurvedic point of view and how best to help the client in further understanding their own mental state.

Physical Constitutions

The following are the ten recognized possible mixes of the three humors—Vata, Pitta, Kapha, Vata/Pitta, Vata/Kapha, Pitta/Vata, Pitta/Kapha, Kapha/Vata, Kapha/Pitta, Vata/Pitta/Kapha.

For massage there is a distinct advantage in using ten rather than seven humor combinations. Pure types constitute about 30% to 40% of my clients. This then leaves the majority of my clients- 60% to 70% of a mixed type. Understanding the difference between a VP person versus a PV person can totally change the way I approach that person and on what type of therapeutic approach I take with them. By adding the mental qualities I can then further pinpoint my approach to the individual concerned. The purpose of this is to give a therapeutic approach that: 1.) achieves a therapeutic action, i.e., heals the person; 2.) that is tailored to the individual; and, 3.) that addresses the person as more than a physical body, i.e., body/mind/soul.

Most books on Ayurveda include a test that helps you to determine your constitution. This book does not include this kind test which is decidedly limited in judging a persons overall nature, not just the physical traits. Instead I have included a chapter on diagnosis to help you determine more precisely your own, and others, constitution. This is something that every therapist should learn anyway and it is much more accurate in understanding your client than the somewhat superficial method of using a questionnaire. A test can be given to people when you are first learning Ayurvedic therapies. However, this should be dispensed with as soon as possible as it will eventually limit your own understanding of the tridosha theory.

There follows a brief description of each of the ten constitutional types. Please note that each constitutional type is also related to one or two of the five pranas (vayu or vata) that govern the body. This information will become clear as you proceed in the book and is extremely important in giving correct treatments.

Vata - Pure vata types are governed by apana-vayu and are of a thin, tall or short frame. They are very sensitive and deep tissue work is usually not appropriate for them. The apana-vayu become easily disturbed in all of the vata types and causes the problems listed below. They are active, irregular, speedy, nervous, tense, have migrating pain, have tendon pain, have muscle pain of sharp nature - usually at a superficial level, they are often deformed or unequal in their body. All of the vata types are cold, usually with poor circulation. They can be very ungrounded in their approach to life and energy. Women will have irregular or difficult menstruation, they may have pre-menstrual difficulties with sharp pain. Emotions can often swing dramatically. Vata types may be prone to accidents.

Vata/Pitta - These persons are governed by both apana and samana-vayu and are more prone to intense migrating pain - at a middle level of muscle - than a pure vata person. In certain cases deep tissue work can be beneficial if the person is well prepared, agrees or even asks for it. They may have a more vata than pitta body. However, be careful about this conclusion as I have noticed about 30% of clients show the opposite body type. Generally, these people will have nervous tension that can become volatile or be expressed in an intense way, yet they will be quite sensitive and require a soft touch. They are prone towards more responsibility than vata types and may suffer from higher levels of stress. Women will have less irregularities than pure vata types, yet will tend to suffer from irregularity and more intense, sharp pain in pre-menstrual times. These people may also be accident prone.

Vata/Kapha - These persons are governed by apana and vyana-vayu and they are more prone to dull migrating pain in deeper tissues. They may have heavy (kapha) bodies even though vata is predominating. This can be discerned by their speech and mental speed. However, they will be very sensitive to touch and one must work slowly into deeper tissues levels than with a pure kapha or other kapha mixes. With proper preparation deep tissue work is acceptable and beneficial. These people can have the tendency to internalize and hold the most nervous stress and tension of the vata types, as with all of the vata predominate types nervousness is high. Women will also tend to suffer from irregularities during menstruation, but with less pain or duller, deeper pain than other types. They are also accident prone or clumsy.

Pitta - Pure pitta types are governed by samana-vayu and are of a middle size and frame. They are more open to touch if they believe the practitioner to be competent and experienced. They will have intense pain localized in one level of muscle, usually the middle tissue level; they will be prone to inflammation of muscles and tissues. Deep tissue work can trigger intense emotions and anger. They should be approached with care and alerted in advance if you feel deeper work is necessary. They are intense people and are active, intelligent, clear, strong willed, dominating, powerful, controlling and decisive. These people are hot in nature and will have good circulation, color and warm hands and feet. Women will often have heavy bleeding and intense local pain during menstruation along with irritability, and intense emotions.

Pitta/Vata - These people are governed by samana and apana-vayu and are hotter than vata/pitta people. They are prone to migrating pain of an intense and sharp nature. Their pain will tend to be localized in one area, yet will migrate more during stressful times. They are prone to have hot, inflamed muscles with underlying nervous tension. They will often be overworked and stressed, resulting in sharp, intense muscle spasms. Women will tend to have irregular, changing cycles with occasional pain and heavy bleeding.

Pitta/Kapha - These people are governed by samana and vyana-vayu and are the coolest of the pitta types with deeper circulation, usually still strong. They will be strong in body and mind and will tend to have powerful muscles. Deep work is generally appropriate at some point during a series of treatments. However, pitta predominate people should always be prepared both mentally and physically before deep penetrating work is done. Muscle pain will tend to be deeper than other pitta types and will be of an intense nature that is constant, deep and localized. Women may have very regular, heavy and long menstruation's with pain during the menses time.

Kapha - Pure kapha types are governed by vyana-vayu and are the strongest and largest of the constitutional types. They are prone to be overweight and slow in their movements and thoughts. They are very stable people and will continue treatments if they understand the need and feel a connection with the practitioner. They are hard to get motivated and changes should be made gradually, yet firmly. They like deep tissue work and will often ask for it on the first session. They love to feel their muscles kneaded and have deposits broken up. Techniques and strokes that use the foot and the flat of the elbow are most appropriate for kapha persons and least (or never) appropriate for vata persons. Pain will tend to be deep, localized and dull in nature. They will be the most attracted to sentimental, deep emotional releases. However, this will only happen when a good relationship exists with the practitioner. They have the slowest circulation and the veins are very deep in the tissues. Women will be very regular in their cycles and have little or no pain. If pain is there it will be of a dull nature. Depression is possible before and during menstruation.

Kapha/Vata - These people are controlled by vyana and apanavayu and are the ones that hold nervous tensions on a deep level. They need deep tissue work, but must be prepared emotionally for it as they are sensitive and usually collect many things in their deep tissues. They must be prepared to let them go during deep work or they will not truly benefit. Fear is often one of the issues present in the deeper tissues. They may have dull migrating pain on a middle or superficial level. They usually have good energy, are interested, and active in life. Stress may play a large role in their body's condition. Their circulation can be the worst of the types (combining irregularity with deep sluggishness). Women may find that their cycles are regular with irregular dull pain some months. Nervous depression may also be present some months.

Kapha/Pitta - These persons are governed by vyana and samana-vayu and are the most active and aggressive of the kapha types. They will tend to have good, deep circulation and large but not overweight bodies. They may have intense pain on a deep level and it tends to be localized. However, it will tend to come only under the stress and strain of work or in emotionally dominating situations. These people are usually not troubled by pain unless undo stress is involved in work or at home. Women will tend to be regular and have trouble free menstruation, perhaps with heavy bleeding or dull aches during the menses.

Secrets of Ayurvedic Massage

Vata/Pitta/Kapha - These people are controlled by the prana-vayu and are said to be larger than pitta, yet smaller than the kapha. They are said to be strong and in good health with no lasting pains or problems. I have never met a person of this constitution so I cannot comment. They are said to be the most rare of the ten types.

It should be pointed out that the prana-vayu is the controlling vayu of the five vayus and is always involved in the health of a person. By the same token, the apana-vayu is always involved in the disease process somehow as it is the opposite of the prana-vayu.

The Sub-Doshas

Each of the three doshas has a subdivision of five aspects, each one controlling a function or system of the body. These are useful to know for a bodyworker as the signs can indicate which dosha is imbalanced. This is not a comprehensive list, but oriented to the massage therapist.

Vata- In general vata controls all movement in the body and mind, it is the principal of movement in nature and in the body. Hence, it relates directly to the nervous system which controls all movement. It relates to the systems of circulation, respiration, muscular movement, motor function, the five senses, evacuation, lactation, menstruation, sexual function, and sweating. Vata is directly related to the bones and bone structure. Vata creates dryness in the body when too high and sluggishness when too low. Together with pitta it controls the hormonal function. The other two humors (doshas) are inert without vata. The five subdivisions control the various aspects of this general description.

Prana vayu- controls inhalation, the other four vayus, the five senses, thinking, health, and proper growth.

Indications of Imbalance- loss of senses, anxiety and worry, insomnia, dryness, emaciation, disease in general.

Apana vayu- controls elimination, sexual function, menstruation, downward movements in the body and disease.

Indications of Imbalance- constipation, menstrual problems, dryness, urinary problems, generally all diseases are involved.

Samana vayu- controls the movement of the digestive system, the solar plexus and balances the prana and apana vayus.

Indications of Imbalance- upset digestion, indigestion, diarrhea, malabsorption of nutrients, dryness.

Udana vayu- controls exhalation, speech, and the upward movements in the body, growth as a child.

Indications of Imbalance- problems of speech and the throat, weakness of will, general fatigue, lack of enthusiasm.

Vyana vayu- pervades the entire body as the nervous system, yet it also controls heart function and circulation of the blood.

Indications of Imbalance- arthritis, nervousness, poor circulation, poor motor reflexes, problems of the joints, bone disorders, nervous disorders.

Pitta- In general pitta is responsible for all metabolic processes in the body. Pitta is the principal of transformation, on both a mental and physical level. Hence, pitta helps us to digest thoughts, feelings and food - or transform them. Pitta controls all heat and heat disorders of the body. Together with vata it controls the hormonal function. Pitta relates to the fiery organs in the body and the blood. It is usually carried by the blood in disturbed states. All inflammations are from excess pitta. Low pitta will cause the whole metabolism to slow down and usually goes with high kapha. Excess pitta causes all kinds of burning and heat related disorders that usually burns up kapha. The five subdivisions control the various aspects of this general description.

Alochaka pitta- controls the ability to see and the digestion of what we see.

Indications of Imbalance- eye problems and difficulties to digest what we see.

Sadaka pitta- controls functions of the heart and the digestion of thoughts and emotions.

Indications of Imbalance- heart failure, repressed emotions and feelings, excessive anger or unprocessed feelings.

Pachaka pitta- controls stomach digestion.

Indications of Imbalance- ulcers, heartburn, cravings, indigestion.

Ranjaka pitta- controls liver / gall bladder digestion.

Indications of Imbalance- anger, irritability, hostility, excessive bile, liver disorders, skin problems, toxic blood, anemia.

Bhrajaka pitta- controls metabolism of the skin.

Indications of Imbalance- all skin problems, acne, inflammation of the skin.

Kapha- In general kapha is responsible for the stability of our body and mind. Kapha is the principal of cohesion in the body and mind. Kapha mainly exists in the body as plasma, blood, muscle and fat tissues. It provides the lubrication and basis for the body. Flexibility and growth are controlled by kapha. Moisture and fluid retention is maintained by this dosha. When kapha is too high it restricts vata and subdues pitta. It creates congestion on all levels of the body. Too little kapha is like high vata, dryness and ungrounded thoughts and actions. The five subdivisions control the various aspects of this general description.

Tarpaka kapha- controls fluids in the head, the sinuses and cerebral fluids.

Indications of Imbalance- sinus problems, headaches, loss of smell.

Bodhaka kapha- controls taste and the cravings of taste, digestion, and saliva.

Indications of Imbalance- overeating and cravings for sweets, loss of taste, congestion in the throat and mouth areas.

Avalambaka kapha- controls lubrication and the fluids around the heart, lungs and upper back.

Indications of Imbalance- congestion in the lungs or heart, stiffness in the back and upper spine, lethargy.

Kledaka kapha- controls the lubrication of the digestive process, maintains a balance with the pitta bile's, provides internal lubrication.

Indications of Imbalance- bloated stomach, slow or congested digestion, excess mucus.

Slesaka kapha- controls the lubrication of the joints in the body and aids in all movements.

Indications of Imbalance- lose joints, swelling joints, stiff joints, painful movements.

Mental Constitutions

In approaching the mental qualities of a person it is important to distinguish between the constitution of the person and the guna that predominates in the mind. Generally, the mental constitution follows the physical. In some cases a person with a pitta/vata constitution will be more vata mentally, then we can say that they are a vata/pitta person. This is because the mind, or total mental functioning, is stronger than the body. Look back on your own life to verify this fact for yourself. How many times have you let a meal go by because you were so interested in something else? Even though your body said it was hungry, you were busy at the time and the body had to wait.

In this way the ten different constitutional types can be used to also determine which humor seems to be stronger in the mind (in the case of mixed constitutions). By putting the humor that is predominate in the mind first - as it is more powerful than the body - the therapist can have an instant clue on how to approach his client.

At this point, once the constitution is determined, the therapist can look at the predominate guna, or quality of the mind. This is an additional factor - yet very important. Below the different types are indicated. This is by no means a comprehensive view, but rather a beginning. The gunas are the most important to see what a client is capable of doing or not doing therapeutically.

The gunas show the basic predisposition of the mentality and what things it values. They indicate the openness of the mind to new ideas or treatments. They are responsible for good or bad habits in health. Too much of tamas, or inactivity, make the mind dull and the body lethargic. Tamas is a natural state in sleep, yet it should be confined to that place and not cultivated in the waking state. Whichever guna is predominating will aid or nullify the therapists treatment. Hence, a thorough understanding of the three gunas is invaluable for any practitioner regardless of the method or practice being used.

A brief description of some of the key words related to the gunas follows:

Sattva - is the quality of peace, happiness, harmony, purity, intelligence, it is clear and has clarity, intuition, knowledge, health.

Rajas - is active, aggressive, dominant, piercing, moving, restless, red, angry, sharp, power orientated, work, action.

Tamas - is dull, slow, dead, lethargic, stupid, violent, perverted, dark, poison, disease, hidden, inertia, sleep.

Life is made up of all three qualities and each is needed in its proper place, such as sleep. The problem arises when tamas or rajas dominate the mentality during the waking state, or when you are awake. Yoga considers pure intelligence to be sattvic in nature, tamas is the opposite of this, or dullness. Rajas is inbetween sattva and tamas. Yoga uses rajas to stimulate tamas and transform it. Rajas is thus used as a step to sattva. Most people today are a mix of rajas and tamas. This is partially due to our diets and our culture with tend to be quite tamasic in nature. What we eat - physically or mentally - ultimately becomes who we are. What we can digest - again mentally and physically - determines what stays in our body /mind /soul.

Sattvic Mentality - The sattvic mind is harmonious and represents a state of mental flexibility. A sattvic person is flexible and responds in the moment to events. They also respond emotionally in accord with the situation. In other words, if you step on my toe, I will not hit you on the head. I will say "Ow, you stepped on my toe!" A sattvic person is open to new things and hold opinions lightly. They are peaceful people and do not get into conflicts. They can be alone or with people. They enjoy nature and their mind is at peace. Hence, they sleep well and are undisturbed by the past or the future. They are well motivated, yet not overly so. They are very trusting, yet have a sharp intuition and intelligence. A sattvic mind is developed through spiritual practice, meditation, prayer and service towards others. A lifestyle that promotes sattva is needed along with a diet that eliminates substances that are rajasic and tamasic.

Rajasic Mentality - The rajasic mind is represented by an active state. A rajasic person tends towards rigid thinking and is very opinionated. They often respond to situations with emotions that are out of context. They are bright and aggressive mentally. They are active and energetic, yet they often lack the ability to stop or slow down. Rajasic people are strongly motivated in life. They usually are always busy at something, they consider rest as 'down time' or a waste. They are often in conflict with people. They like to use things and think a lot. Rajasic people can do any step needed to heal themselves if they are sure it will benefit them and not waste time and energy. They are good at motivating others, but often lack discretion in how this can be used. Their sleep is often disturbed and they have difficulty to turn off their thinking process.

Tamasic Mentality - The tamasic mind is represented by a stagnant state. A tamasic person is dull witted or lacking in intelligence. They are not motivated and cannot do anything without pressure or force from someplace (it can be that they force themselves). They over sleep, over indulge and are prone to excess in all forms. They are often depressed or down emotionally. They can drain those around them and become undesirable company. Tamasic people are thieves, murderers or those who exploit others. They are associated with vice in all forms and with drugs. All pharmaceutical products are tamasic in quality and so make the mind tamasic. Tamasic people eat junk and processed foods. Meat and alcohol are tamasic in nature and bring violence and dullness to the mind. They are lethargic and incapable of appreciating beauty in life. They are often obsessed with money or sexual gratification. Tamasic people have no real opinions, they follow the masses and what is popular. They make poor clients and usually will be brought to a therapist and seldom, if ever, come on their own. Thus, any form of treatment with a tamasic

Secrets of Ayurvedic Massage

person is difficult unless rajas exists in enough quantity to bring change.

While reviewing this information use common sense. If someone is tamasic in nature it can mean that they are self destructive and chronically depressed. It does not necessarily mean that every tamasic person is a drug dealer that murders people. By the same token, every rajasic person is not a power hungry politician (although all power hungry politicians are rajasic!).

Usually, people are made up of all three to some extent. In our culture sattvic people are rare. As a professional health care therapist you will be dealing with rajasic mixes of people - i.e., mixed with sattva or tamas. True tamasic people will not come to you. They might, however, rob you on your way home!

The instances in my practice where people have not benefited have been those cases where someone has forced another one to come and see me. I generally do not accept to work with someone unless two conditions are met: 1.) they come of their own accord (i.e., they want to get well) and 2.) they pay me for it (i.e., they value it). These two conditions indicate that there is enough rajas for the therapy to succeed. If one of these conditions is not met it indicates a predominance of tamas and success will be difficult. Allopathic (Western medicine) is better suited to people of a tamasic nature as they are not ready to accept responsibility for their own health.

There is no judgment in these observations - it is a simple vision of how people function. Massage therapy or any form of natural healing is not for everyone. Understanding the three gunas and how they function gives a therapist the tools to help people according to their capacity. In some cases it may actually benefit persons more to recommend them to a normal doctor than to pursue natural therapies that they are unable to perform.

---

[1] Atreya, *Practical Ayurveda: Secrets of Physical, Sexual & Spiritual Health*, York Beach, Me; Samuel Weiser, Inc. 1998

[2] Dr. Robert Svoboda, *Prakruti; Your Ayurvedic Constitution*, Albuquerque, NM; Geocom, Ltd. 1989

2 The Importance of Prana in Ayurvedic Massage

"From a combination of the rajas portions of the five subtle elements arose the prana. Again, due to difference of function it is divided into five."

—Pancadasi, I-22

The secret of Ayurveda, and thus of Ayurvedic massage, is Prana. In fact Ayurvedic medicine is the science of prana. If a practitioner understands the power of prana, its functions, its currents, its junctions and manifestations then that person holds not only the secrets of massage, but of all natural healing. Ultimately, it is the prana that a therapist is working on, in massage or otherwise.

This knowledge is not easily found or given. However difficult this information is to find it is even more difficult to really understand it. I have been teaching the secrets of prana for many years and not one of my students really understands yet that the divine *is* Prana. If you befriend this Prana it will do everything for you. If you honor this Prana it will help you. If you worship this Prana it will carry you to the other shore.

What Is Prana?

Sometimes the impossible must be attempted in order to expand the horizons of mankind. It is with this in mind that I attempt to explain *prana*. The reason for this is that prana is synonymous with life. Without it nothing lives, breaths or moves. One can say that living is prana and that life is prana.

15

In one respect it is possible to understand life in a physical or mundane sense and on another level it is completely unknowable and mysterious. It is the second that I wish to address first, even though it is the physical that we shall finally use in the techniques presented here. The purpose of this is twofold; first, it is done this way in the tradition that I follow, and secondly, it is necessary for massage to be used as a true healing therapy.

The first teacher I had in massage, Swami Ananda, understood the mystery of prana. To this day, more than twelve years later, I have yet to meet another person who had such a touch. Whenever he would speak about prana tears would come to his eyes and he would have to stop speaking because he was so overwhelmed by emotion. As the years have gone by I too have come to love this profoundness that the ancients called prana. The Sanskrit word *prana* means 'primal energy'; pra = before, ana = breath or the energy of breathing; life. To understand the mystery of prana is to understand the mystery of life.

I have explained at some length prana and have even compared it to the Chinese concept of Chi in *Practical Ayurveda*. In essence people who say that chi or ki are different than prana have not penetrated the mystery of any of them. The mind loves to divide and categorize. First, there is intellectual understanding which is the most divisional and is the most superficial. When this understanding becomes experiential rather than intellectual a second level of division is present; less, yet still making differences. At some point the experiential stops and a practitioner becomes 'one with' or merged into the work. In this understanding there is no difference of Chi or Prana. Statements that reflect divisions are indicative of the persons development, not the reality of energy in its subtle form.

Prana is both manifest and un-manifest energy; *Purusha* and Prakruti. The two great cosmic forces that are the cause of manifestation in the ancient view of creation. In its un-manifest state it is the energy of consciousness (purusha-shakti). In its manifest form it is the energy of creation (prakruti-shakti). These two aspects follow prana throughout its many later expressions. One is always the conscious side and the other the active or material side. In the body we perceive these two as the movement of thought in consciousness, or as the instinctive intelligent function of the metabolism. Hence, prana is at the very root of creation and nothing can exist without it.

A sage was sitting in meditation and went into a super-conscious state (*samadhi*). He lost body contact and his spirit merged with the un-manifest consciousness. His body was sitting still and straight in a yoga posture. As time went on his body slowly began to deteriorate and decompose. Bugs and animals ate parts of the body and the elements slowly destroyed the flesh as the years passed. One day the sage had a slight movement of self awareness and he found himself regaining bodily awareness. However, his body was by now a dried bag of decomposed bones and skin. As his consciousness returned so did the vital force; the prana. When his awareness fully awakened and returned his body was the same as when he had left it - young and healthy.

This ancient story shows the deep relationship that prana has with the soul. As long as the soul has not relinquished its hold on the body, it cannot die. Thus the yogi was able to rest in cosmic consciousness and the body did not 'die'. The relationship of the body to the soul is due to the prana. In this way it is often called the 'life-force' because when the soul departs the prana or life-force goes too. In the above story it was not a good thing because it thwarted the sages efforts of many years. It illustrates that he was not completely pure in his re-identification to the cosmic being and was so pulled back by the idea of a physical separateness. Often prana is called the soul.

Traditionally there are two means to find the source of both the manifest and un-manifest. One is to follow the currents of thoughts back to their source and the other is to follow the prana back to its source. Working with prana can be *Yoga* - union with the divine. The mind also can lead one to Yoga. The secret to both of these methods is to know that there is a substratum that is before, or prior to, the manifest and un-manifest.

Here it is necessary to give a definition of what is meant by 'mind' in the Vedic sense. Mind is not a concrete substance, it is made up of several different subtle components and the sum total of these we call 'mind'. The first level is intellect, your reasoning ability. Second, is your unconscious mind, that which holds emotions and impressions. Thirdly, there is the basic intelligence that provides the basis for the other two and carries memories.

Lastly, there is a pure field of awareness in which all of the others exist. It is this last one which is considered to be the sattvic mind in Yoga and Ayurveda. In this book all of the above four layers comprise the 'mind'.

Within the context of using the above two methods to find the source of either mind or prana, there are two additional methods - force or friendship; will or worship; control or communion; power or pleasing. The way of the yogi or of the martial artist is of power, or control. The way of the healer is to befriend, to worship, to be in communion with that force which is the source of life itself.

The same is true with the mind. You can try control or friendship with the mind. In respect to both prana and mind the way of control is the most uncertain. You may or may not succeed. If your will is strong you may, with time, be able to control the movement of mind or the movement of prana. In any case this is a lifetime work and twenty years is a normal period of time for a person to practice and master their chosen art.

As a practitioner I am sure that you are reading this to find secrets to add rather quickly to your practice. This is why I am proposing the alternative approach to the classical yogic method of control - at least as understood in the West. *Bhakti Yoga*, or devotion, is the alternative means. If you are befriended by this Power you are sure to achieve the same results - and I feel better - than through the method of will power. The certainty of success is guaranteed if you are sincere (once you actually 'touch' the prana this is not difficult as it is so beautiful). Not only that but by a communion with the prana you are actually communing with 'life'. This is extremely important as a healing practitioner. As a healthcare professional your attitude towards life is all important. If it is life positive then your work will be a success and your clients will be healed. If your attitude is life negative it will reflect in a loss of clients, poor results and personal periods of depression.

Hence, one of the main 'secrets' of prana is to cultivate a strong communion with her. If you are friends with someone you help them. This is the definition of friendship. The prana will befriend you if you allow it by having the right attitude. The 'right attitude' is traditionally called devotion. As this word has a negative connotation to the individualistic ego orientated society

18   *Secrets of Ayurvedic Massage*

that we live in I have to use the word communion. In essence it is the same. Another way to say it is a sense of awe or wonder that the prana inspires. Cultivate this sense of wonder or mystery and that, coupled with honor and respect, is devotion to the Western person. This at least is a good beginning. True devotion comes naturally with time to a sincere person.

I guarantee that if you follow this advise your work will improve dramatically. Like real friendships your relation to prana will deepen over time. This deepening will be reflected in the quality of your work and the well-being of your patients.

"He who adores the prana and the apana thus is not reborn in this world again and he is freed from all bondage."[1]

On the physical level of the body prana is understood as the vitality or life force that animates the organism. This is primarily done by its movement through the nadis or meridians. The movement of prana in the nadis is facilitated by the material manifestation of the chakras. These 'chakras' are not and have nothing to do with the subtle chakras that are related to changes in consciousness.

Please excuse me if I repeat some items here about chakras that I have covered in another book[2], it is nonetheless important. There is a basic misunderstanding about the chakras of the Yogic tradition. This misunderstanding can be traced back to the turn of the century and the Theosophical Society. Their information on the chakras and other aspects of the yogic subtle anatomy are absolutely not in keeping with the ancient tradition of Yoga. This has caused a basic misunderstanding and has been amplified by 'new age' groups throughout the West. If one takes the time to read the ancient scriptures the discrepancy is clear. The primary misunderstanding is that of the chakras as a vehicle for physical changes versus that of changes in consciousness. It is the physical and energetic application of the chakras that we, as massage therapists, are concerned with. It is the realm of Kundalini Yoga to develop chakras as vehicles for uplifting consciousness.

According to the Yogic scriptures humanity is not given these subtle chakras that work on consciousness directly - one has to develop them through spiritual practice. Their 'physical' (actually etheric) counterparts have nothing to do with the 'consciousness' of a person. They are simply "pumping stations" of pranic energy through the nadis. Hence, when alternative practitioners talk about 'opening chakras' and such they are referring (whether they know it or not) to the physical centers. These are also the centers that clairvoyants see with their subtle vision. This information is well documented in the Yogic scriptures of India and is thousands of years old. It is only a recent phenomenon that some confusion exists in the West about the chakras.

While it is not my intention to harp over this point it is important that we compare apples to apples and not oranges and apples. In Ayurveda and Yoga a chakra is used in the context of 'consciousness' only as applied to Kundalini Yoga or Laya Yoga (the Yoga of Fusion). Kriya Yoga can also be used in this fashion. Understand that these methods are lifetime methods and that one cannot achieve results in a couple of years. An excellent reference in this regard is the book *Tantric Yoga* [3]. All other references in Ayurveda and other branches of yoga are considering chakras as a kind of marma, sensitive points of pranic energy, that help in the circulation and distribution of prana through the nadis (see fig. 1).

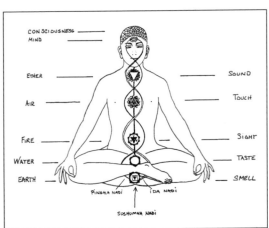

Fig. 1

Prana and the Mind

Prana and the mind are so closely entwined together that it is impossible to separate them. To speak about prana is ultimately to speak about pure intelligence, or sattvic mind. They are two sides of the same coin. Without prana there is no movement in consciousness, without intelligence there is no direction to the movement. The two operate together at all times. Thus the methods mentioned above are complimentary. Even if you think you are only working on the prana, the mind will also be effected, and vice versa.

The great Vedic seer Vasistha describes this relationship-

"By control of the life-force the mind is also restrained; even as the shadow ceases when the substance is removed, the mind ceases when the life-force is restrained."[4]

The analogy of the shadow and form is used again and again in Vedic literature to indicate that prana is the shadow of the Source, the Self, the Formless that Purusha and Prakruti arise from. The mind is then led to the Source by the prana as indicated by the ancient scripture, *Prasna Upanishad*.

"From the Self is born this Prana. Just as there can be the shadow when a man is there, so this Prana is fixed on the Self. He comes to this body owing to the actions of the mind."[5]

This understanding is necessary to work effectively with the human body. You are not working with a mass of ligaments, tissues, organs and plasma. You are working with the Divine in a sentient form. Always remember this, even if your client does not.

Description of the Five Pranas

Prana divides five fold in the body to support all movement and bodily functions. It is this five fold division that is related to vata, the humor of movement in Ayurveda. Vata has been described as prana that is outward moving. When prana is kept internalized as in spiritual practices or meditation it is healthy and in a potent, latent form. When it begins to move outward through the senses and mind it becomes vata.

Each of the three humors has a refined state or a potent, subtle state. The subtle state of pitta is *Tejas* and the subtle state of kapha is *Ojas*. Once more this is described very precisely in Dr. Frawley's *Tantric Yoga* as cited above. One can heal the body by developing these subtle forms of the three humors. It is more properly a yogic alchemical process and not something to play with. Normally the humors cause disease in their excess states. Yet to develop more Prana, Tejas and Ojas the humors must be in equal excess - this is difficult to accomplish without discipline and clear guidance.

The five pranas are normally called the five vayus. Hence we will describe them as such to avoid confusion as the chief among them is also called prana, although it is different than the cosmic prana that the sub vayus are derived from. Look at the description in Chapter One of the five sub-doshas of vata to further clarify the comprehensive role that the five vayus play in the body and mind.

Prana vayu is the 'foreword or inward moving air' as it moves inward and receives all impressions into the body. It is located in the head and heart; controls thinking, inhalation, emotions, the sensory functioning, memory, and receiving cosmic prana from the sun; hot or solar prana. It provides the basic energy that moves us in life. Strong prana is the source of health.

Apana vayu is the 'downward moving air' as it moves down and outward. It is seated in the colon and controls all the processes of elimination including urine, sweat, menstruation, orgasm and defecation. The apana receives cosmic prana from the earth and moon; cool or lunar prana. It also rules the elimination of negative emotions and provides mental stability. It is the basis of our immune system and when disturbed is behind the cause of most diseases.

Udana vayu is called the 'upward moving air' as it moves up the spine to reconnect us to the divine. It is located in the throat; controls speech, connects us to the solar and lunar forces (sky and earth; masculine and feminine) and is responsible for all spiritual development. Udana controls psychic powers and psychic phenomena, and controls creative expression. The development of the kundalini relates directly to the udana prana. It governs growth of the body.

Samana vayu is called the 'equalizing or balancing air' and it moves from the periphery to the center. It is seated in the navel and controls the digestive system and harmonizes prana and apana. Samana also governs the digestion of air, of emotions and feelings. It is hot and solar in nature. What sumana digests becomes the vyana vayu.

Vyana vayu is called the 'pervading or outward moving air' as it moves from the center to the periphery. It is seated in the heart, yet pervades the whole body. It unites the other pranas and the tissues and controls nerve and muscle action. It holds the body together. It is responsible for all circulation in the body; food, blood, and emotions. Vyana provides strength and stability to the body.

Additionally, there are five more minor pranas or vayus. They are called Naga, Kurma, Krkara, Devadatta, and Dhanamjaya. They control the following actions specifically: Hiccuping, opening and closing the eyes, digestion, yawning, and the vayu that stays after death, still holding the body together.

This description of the five main vayus (five pranas) is not definitive. They interrelate to each other and are very complex in their movements and relationships. Consider this a beginning. Use it to begin to understand - by experience - your own movement of prana. This is felt by first becoming aware of your breath. When breath awareness is there then awareness of prana will follow. Do not except my word for this - do it and feel the differences in your own body in meditation. You must be aware of your own prana before you can be aware of someone else's prana.

[1] *Yoga Vasistha, "The Supreme Yoga"* Vols. I & II, Swami Venkatesananda trans., Shivanandanagar, Uttar Pradesh, India: Divine Life Society, 1991, Vol. I, pg. 367

[2] Atreya, *Prana: The Secret of Yogic Healing*, York Beach, ME; Samuel Weiser, 1996, chapter 10

[3] Frawley, Dr. David, *Tantric Yoga and the Wisdom Goddesses*, Salt Lake City, UT: Passage Press, 1994

[4] *Yoga Vasistha, "The Supreme Yoga"* Swami Venkatesananda trans., Shivanandanagar, Uttar Pradesh, India: Divine Life Society, 1991, page 229, vol. I

[5] Eight Upanishads, trans. Swami Gambhirananda, Calcutta, India: Advaita Ashrama, 1992 Vol. II, page 439

3 The Place of Meditation In Ayurvedic Therapies

"When the mind gradually leaves off the ideas of the meditator and the act of meditation and is merged in the sole object of meditation (the Self), and is steady like the flame of a lamp in a breezeless spot; it is called the super conscious state (samadhi)."

—Pancadasi, I-55

The place of meditation in the healing arts cannot be underestimated. This is due to one fundamental law of the universe - you cannot give what you don't have. There is a beautiful story of Mahatma Ghandi in this regard.

A woman brought her child to the Mahatma for his help. After inquiring what the problem was the mother told him, 'Please tell my child to stop eating sugar as he is diabetic and it will cause him harm'. Ghandi told her to come back in a week. When the two returned a week later Ghandi told the child to stop eating sugar. The mother then asked him, 'Why didn't you tell him that last week and save us the journey to come back again?'. Ghandi replied, 'Last week I was still eating sugar'.

As a therapist you must be of a certain development or your clients will be effected by your state. The more refined your energy system and mind are the better work you will be able to do and the broader base of a clientele you will be able to touch. A coarse mind and energy system will attract a similar kind of person. A more refined mind and energy system will attract a more refined clientele, yet these people can also treat successfully the less refined. A client who has done internal work will feel bad from a technically good masseur if that practitioner has not done any work on themselves. Let me illustrate this with a personal experience.

Some years ago I was went to a bodyworker that was new in the ashram that I lived. He was reputed to have a 'soft touch'. As I have a degenerating condition in my spine, coupled with ky-phoscoliosis, I was usually uncomfortable with deep work (although I have had several series of deep tissue work that helped me tremendously, it is simply not appropriate for the maintenance of my body). The masseur was a young man in his twenties and after asking a few questions and us talking a bit he began to work. Almost as soon as he started to work on me I began to feel bad. I could literally feel his 'junk' flowing down his arms into my body. What he was doing was technically correct, yet he was neither mentally present nor conscious of what was going on. By the end of an hour I felt sick and very uncomfortable in my body. The feeling I had was that I had done the healing, not him. Have you ever felt this after a session? I know several people who have had this experience, I believe it to be fairly common.

Of course, I should have gotten up and stopped the session, but I was also just learning bodywork at the time and didn't really understand what was happening. His prana was flowing into me - as it does with every bodyworker - and carried his mental state with it. This is the law explained in the previous chapter - mind and prana always function together. The result was that I went for a session to feel better and ended up feeling worse.

What should be explained to put this into context is that I had been meditating daily for nine or ten years at that time. I began to meditate at the age of 17 and continued sitting until I was 34 when I met my present Guru. The young man who had worked on me had obviously not done any or little internal work.

Through the teaching of my Guru I learned that true meditation had not happened to me after seventeen years of sitting (or often trying to sit!). During most of those years I was working and had a family, so it was difficult to find time each day. I ending up rising at 5 or 5:30 each morning so that I could have some time to myself. I must say that the first years were filled with frustration and the seeming lack of progress. However, slowly,

Secrets of Ayurvedic Massage

and in spite of many stops and starts, a certain equilibrium was achieved. At the time of this story I was doing the Buddhist meditation of Vipassana and continued to do so for the next five years. When I finally understood what meditation was I had tried numerous methods and had achieved a frame of mind that felt quite peaceful.

I understood after many conversations with my Guru that what I was doing all those years was a practice and not *Dhyana*, or meditation. My mentor explained that a subtle trinity existed in all techniques and practices that actually kept the one doing the exercises in a confined state; i.e., not achieving the goal of meditation - peace of mind or union with the divine - that is actually the source of all peace. In the act of meditating there is the one doing it, the action of it, and the object being focused on. I found out that this is explained beautifully in a little book called *Tripura Rahasya*, or *The Mystery Beyond the Trinity*.[1] This explanation and the study of different scriptures like the one above and the *Yoga Vasistha* [2] helped me to realize that meditation is a *state of being* that has nothing to do with the 'mind' as described in Chapter Two.

It is this approach that we must bring into our work as practitioners - our 'state of being'. All methods and practice help to develop this. However, true meditation is a 24 hour affair that is not done - it is lived. Living whatever your state of being is is your *Dharma* or path in life. One can refine their state of being by hatha yoga, pranayama, vipassana, mantra, japa, and many other forms of practice. Meditation is none of these things. It is a flowering of your maturity. This flowering results in a refined state of being. In Ayurveda this is called a sattvic mind. The divine can only reveal itself to a sattvic mind.

Of what concern is this to a massage therapist? First, it will allow a beautiful quality of prana to flow into your patients. Second, it is this state of being that - carried by the prana - heals the same latent state of being in the client. Or, as in the example given above, the reverse can also happen. If you are angry, that anger passes into the others that you touch, whether you know it or not. Third, true healing happens only when the 'state of being' is touched in the patient. Last, you become a happier and more peaceful person.

Hence, if one wishes to practice Ayurvedic massage, one must be willing to touch more than the body. Ayurveda is a mind / body system of medicine. The only way to effectively change the mental state - or help create the possibility of change - in another is by letting your own state encompass them. The mingling of these two will create an alchemy that effects a change. You cannot touch the deep levels of consciousness in another if you have not dived into your own depths.

Stored Impressions

"Wherever it roams in space, the jiva (soul), which is of the nature of prana or life-force, sees whatever forms are conjured up by its previous vasanas or impressions. These previous impressions are destroyed only by intense self-effort. Even if the mountains were pulverized and the worlds dissolved, one should not give up self-effort. Even heaven and hell are but the projections of these impressions or vasanas."[3]

Stored impression in the bodies - physical, energetic, emotional, mental, and casual - are called *Vasanas* and *Samskaras* in the Vedic tradition. All bodyworkers are aware of stored impressions that exist in the muscle tissues and in deep connective tissues. The release of these as a therapeutic method is well documented in other works and it is not the purpose of this book to explain the therapeutic value of releasing these stored impressions. It is, however, the purpose of this book to put it into the correct context of Ayurveda.

An excellent view of how to incorporate this kind of work into an Ayurvedic practice is presented in *Ayurveda & Life Impressions Bodywork*.[4] This is a good book on the subject and should be read by persons wishing to do bodywork from an Ayurvedic, though not traditional, point of view.

In the Vedic tradition these impressions are the cause of all disease. I have explained this in great detail in *Practical Ayurveda* and also in *Prana: The Secret of Yogic Healing*, so there is no need to go into the subject again. The elimination of these impressions is necessary for health and for spiritual development. In fact, subtle development can only happen with the dissolving of vasanas and samskaras. Vasanas are impressions that are latent and are carried from body to body, life to life until they have opportunity to be liberated by letting them arise and disappear. They are deeper than the unconscious mind and have no relation to it. They are the forces that propel us in life to become - say, a politician - heaven forbid!

> "He who is able to abandon this vasana while yet living in the body in this world is said to be liberated. He who has not abandoned vasana is in bondage, even if he is a great scholar."[5]

Samskaras are the impressions that are accumulated in this life (vasanas are also constantly being accumulated) and are the impressions that relate to the unconscious or subconscious mind. They are the ones that are activated and - hopefully - liberated in bodywork.

> "Consciousness has the faculty of holding on to something; a notion so held is known as samskara. But when it is realized that the notion is only reflected in consciousness, it is seen that there is no samskara independent of consciousness."[6]

Both samskaras and vasanas are held in all the bodies, depending on what kind of thought, emotion or action formed them. They are usually concentrated around marmas or chakras, even in the subtle bodies. In Kundalini Yoga it is the vasanas that form the 'knots' at each center that must be cleared and liberated for the *Shakti* (prana) to rise.

It is part of the function of Ayurvedic bodywork to liberate the samskaras. This can only be accomplished by two prerequisites being met: 1.) the practitioner must have a refined state of being that is the result of their own interior work, and 2.) there must be no preconceived idea or concept of healing or helping the other.

As long as the practitioner carries any idea of helping another then he or she is trapped in the trinity mentioned above. It is the elimination of concepts that defines what meditation is, Dhyana. If you can work without any concept of what you are doing - and this does not mean your actual technique, it means the position of your mind, not your hands - then true healing happens naturally. True healing is the union of the Cosmic Being with the Individualized being of the client. The therapist can in fact do nothing. He or she can act as a catalyst for the cosmic being to touch the individualized being. This is the purpose and function of meditation in Ayurvedic therapies.

Exercises

The following exercises are not meditations, however, they can eventually lead one to meditation. They are all specifically beneficial for bodyworkers. They activate the pranas and clear and open the nadis. All breathing is done through the nose, equal breathing in both nostrils if possible. If one nostril is plugged, do not worry, it will either clear or there is a reason for it to be closed. Refer to Chapter Five for an explanation to the nadis.

Exercise One- Sit in a relaxed position, on the floor or in a chair. Breath a few times deeply and in a relaxed manner. Now place your hands on your lower abdomen, holding your belly. Breath in slowly and feel your belly move out slightly. As your lungs fill up with air they push the diaphragm down, causing your lower abdomen to move out slightly. Exhale in a relaxed manner, without tension, yet slowly. The exhale should be slightly longer than the inhale.

As you breath in simply put your attention on your hands, don't worry or think about the breath. By putting your attention on your hands, i.e., the belly, the prana -via the breath - will go there. As you exhale simply allow the air to flow from your nostrils. In other words, focus your attention on the nostrils and don't think about the breath. In all of these exercises it is easier to focus on the final point or destination of the breath than to work directly on the breath itself.

Repeat this rhythmical breathing for 5 - 15 minutes, once or twice per day, especially before or between sessions.

Benefit - This exercise charges your body with prana (meaning in this sense, all five of the vayus), it creates a reservoir of energy that helps to maintain your own pranic level while you work. It opens and clears the three main nadis in the body, facilitating your own health, purity, and mental clarity. By energizing the three main nadis all of the other nadis are effected to some degree.

Exercise Two- Sit in a relaxed position, on the floor or in a chair. This is a continuation of exercise one adding another step to the inhalation and the exhalation. Breath into your lower abdomen until you feel your hands move out slightly. Then continue to breath in but now direct your breath upwards to the heart area. Hold the breath there for an instant and then exhale slowly with your attention on your hands. Feel the breath (i.e., prana via the breath) go out of your hands.

As you breath in feel the prana enter into your belly and then travel upwards to your heart area. Once there allow it to flow out through your hands. You may use a visual picture of white or golden light as the prana flowing into your body and out of your hands. In this method you are consciously opening and using the *Yashasvati* and *Hastijihva* nadis that govern the movement of the arms and legs, terminating in the palms of the hands and the soles of the feet. As you hold the breath in the heart area for an instant, so too the breath should be held before inhaling again. This is called full and empty retention of breath (*kumbaka*). They should always be equal in duration.

Repeat this exercise for 10 minutes each day, especially before giving any kind of bodywork session.

Benefit - This exercise works like the first exercise but adds these additional benefits: it charges the first three chakras and opens the fourth; it opens the nadis of the arms and hands, increasing your sensitivity and ability to transmit healing prana to the client; it allows you to feel on a more subtle level the state of your client; it helps develop your ability to take pulse and use Ayurvedic diagnostic methods; it helps to center your work in the heart or center you in a space of unconditional giving - this facilitates your work; it brings you peace of mind and body.

Exercise Three- This exercise is an advanced exercise and should not be done unless you are proficient in the above exercises or in pranayama. In any case *this exercise should not be done more than* *five minutes per day without exception*, regardless of your previous experience. Failure to heed this advise will certainly result in an imbalance in your energetic system and will cause, in one form or another, some psychological or physiological disease. However, if done as prescribed it is safe and an amazingly effective method.

Sit in a chair or on the floor in a relaxed position. Take a few normal breaths to relax and get comfortable. You may want to do five minutes or so of exercise number two to get focused on your breath. Fix your eyes on the space between your eyebrows and visualize the incoming breath as white light. Keep your eyes fixed on this point (between the eyebrows) for the duration of the five minute exercise. Your eyes should not be strained, they should be relaxed, yet fixed on the point you choose. Try several points higher or lower on your forehead to find a relaxed point to fix your gaze. Your eyes should be neither closed, nor open, but half open and unfocused.

Breath into your lower abdomen until you feel the hands resting on your belly move slightly outwards. Visualize this as white light. At this moment continue to inhale the breath (prana) up your spinal column until it reaches the top of your head; hold it there for a moment. See the top of your head filled with white light.

Now see this white light pour forth from the top of your head as a fountain and pour around your body, falling to the floor. Like you are under a shower of light. This is done on the exhalation. Remain with empty lungs for a moment before inhaling the next breath. The moment of breath retention should be equal with full lungs (i.e., light filling the top of the head) and with empty lungs (i.e., after exhalation and before inhalation).

Repeat this exercise over and over for five minutes per day. Under no circumstances is it recommended to do for longer periods. It will take several try's before you become proficient.

Benefit - Gives all the benefits of the two previous exercises plus it cleanses all nadis and chakras; purifies the mind; purifies the etheric and astral bodies (the subtle body in Yoga); increase health and immune function; strengthens the physical body; increases prana and tejas in the body.

[1] Ramanananda, Swami, *Tripura Rahasya*, Tiruvannamalai, India: Sri Ramanasramam, 1989

[2] *Yoga Vasistha*, *"The Supreme Yoga"* Swami Venkatesananda trans., Shivanandanagar, Uttar Pradesh, India: Divine Life Society, 1991

[3] *Yoga Vasistha*, *"The Supreme Yoga"* Swami Venkatesananda trans., Shivanandanagar, Uttar Pradesh, India: Divine Life Society, 1991 Vol. II pg. 414

[4] Vanhowten, Donald, *Ayurveda & Life Impressions Bodywork*, Twin Lakes, WI; Lotus Press, 1997

[5] *Yoga Vasistha*, *"The Supreme Yoga"* Swami Venkatesananda trans., Shivanandanagar, Uttar Pradesh, India: Divine Life Society, 1991 Vol. II pg. 414

[6] *Yoga Vasistha*, *"The Supreme Yoga"* Swami Venkatesananda trans., Shivanandanagar, Uttar Pradesh, India: Divine Life Society, 1991 Vol. II pg. 648

4 Diagnostic Methods

"The mind, the ruler of the ten organs of sense and action,
is situated within the lotus of the heart. As it depends on
the organs of sense and action for its functions in relation
to external objects, it is called an internal organ."
—Pancadasi, II-12

A king was riding with his court through the forest when they came across a naked man sitting under a tree laughing. They rode on a little way until the king ordered everyone to stop. He was intrigued by the happiness of the man. The king reflected: 'I am a king and I am not really happy. Why is this man so happy?' Thinking thus he sent his messenger to the naked man to tell him to come before the king. The naked one continued to laugh and completely ignored the messenger. The messenger returned to the king with empty hands and related what happened.

The king was an intelligent man and realized that the naked man must be a holy saint lost in the bliss of the divine - who else would dare to disobey his orders? Considering all this in his mind he went alone to the man and asked him, 'What has made you so happy? Who is your Guru? Please tell me so that I can also go to this teacher and find the same bliss'. The naked man stopped laughing and looked deeply at the king and said, 'I have had 24 gurus, a bird has taught me, a young boy, the sky, the rain, a dog, and a snake. I have learned from everything around me, life is my Guru.' So saying he began once more to laugh, overwhelmed by the bliss of the divine.

Diagnosis is like this - learn from everyone and everything. Take all things into consideration when you meet a client. Begin by looking at them - really looking. What kind of body do they have? What kind of face? Hair? Skin? Eyes? These will help to tell you the basic constitution. Then talk to them, ask questions. How do they respond? What kind of mind do they have? Fast? Slow? In-between? Are they excited? What guna is predominating? Are they up? Are they depressed? Did they come of their own accord? Did someone push them to come? Do they feel open? Speaking and listening can tell you everything about a client if you are quiet and understand the three humors well in conjunction with the three gunas. This should provide the basis of your diagnosis.

To know the natal constitution of the client (prakruti) and then to be able to know the current constitution, or imbalance state (vakruti) is the object of diagnosis. This can be done in a simple manner or in a very sophisticated way. This depends on the skill and ability of the therapist. All variations exist in the Ayurvedic system. As a massage therapist you should learn the basics outlined in this chapter, if not immediately, then progressively.

The importance of diagnosis in any form of Ayurvedic therapy is extremely important. While there is a mystic around such forms of diagnosis as pulse, several doctors are helping to dispel the aura of supernatural or extraordinary abilities needed to successfully diagnose a patient. Dr. Vasant Lad is the notable leader in this field of presenting a clear systematic method to read pulse.[1] His works should be studied by all serious students of Ayurveda. I personally follow his method and find it to be quite effective and accurate.

In the basic level diagnosis means understanding the constitution of the person to be treated. The ability to discern the prakruti is of paramount importance in implementing the correct kind of massage. Traditionally, this responsibility rested on the doctor in charge, not the massage therapist. As times have changed this responsibility now rests on the therapist.

Talking with your client is one of the most important methods of diagnosis. By talking to them you can see if they are nervous, or anxious. You can discern which of the three gunas is predominating by their responses to your questions. Questioning itself is invaluable. I usually look at their tongue and take their pulse before I begin asking questions. First, I am not influenced by their problems, and second, I can often find the problem before they tell me of it. This inspires confidence in your professionalism. This also enables you to ask the right questions to further define the type and nature of the person (prakruti) and their imbalance (vakruti).

Pulse

In modern India pulse diagnosis is no longer taught as part of the national curriculum in the university system. This indicates two things: 1.) that it is not necessary to know pulse to treat people effectively in the Ayurvedic system, and; 2.) a horrible mistake is present in the Ayurvedic education system in India.

I personally know of three different methods of pulse diagnosis being used in India at the present and I believe that others exist as well. It is this difference in approaches that has caused pulse diagnosis to be dropped from the curriculum in the university system. My experience is that all three of the systems work well, it is more a question of the practitioner than of the method. This again refers back to the personal development of the therapist and the importance of meditation. All forms of meditation or practice are helpful in developing the skill of pulse diagnosis.

In fact taking the pulse is a meditation. The first prerequisite is for the therapist to be calm and internally quiet (all spiritual practices help create this quiet). Secondly, the therapist must not have stimulated his own pranas - the five vayus - in any manner. This means the eight forbidden actions before taking pulse - for the patient as well as the therapist. They are: 1.) after eating or drinking alcohol or other stimulants like coffee and black tea; 2.) after sunbathing; 3.) after massage; 4.) after sitting next to a source of heat or cooking over the stove; 5.) after hard exercise; 6.) when hungry; 7.) after sex; and 8.) after a bath or shower.

The next important thing to be aware of is your own receptivity. This infers two things - your pranic state and your mental state. If both are quiet and not moving much your receptivity will be higher. The art of taking pulse relies first on *the ability of the therapist to not have any opinion prior to taking the pulse*. If the therapist approaches the patient with a preconceived idea it will actually change the pulse of the person that you are taking. Your own prana will pass into the patient and help create your preconception.

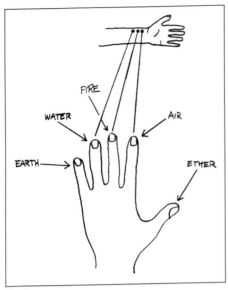

Fig. 2

For example, if a large person (almost fat) comes to me and before taking pulse I am convinced that he or she is kapha in nature, it will help to influence their pulse rate accordingly. The person may have a kapha vakruti (imbalance) and actually be a vata person with low, congested vata. Hence, exhibiting kapha traits. Be relaxed and open with your clients and go through the methods outlined here before coming to a conclusion. This is the correct procedure in diagnosis. Add the sum total of several different techniques to come up with a result.

In this book I will not go into detail as in *Practical Ayurveda* about the differences of pulse. Rather the focus is on what a massage therapist should know before beginning their session. This is the ability to first find the patients prakruti and secondly to determine the patients vakruti.

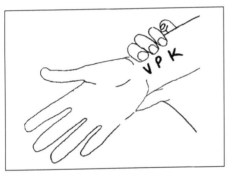

Fig. 3

Prakruti is known by the location, speed, depth, quality, and which part of the finger it hits. Vakruti is known by location, speed, quality and depth. As my father told me many times: "Son, there are three things important in Real Estate; Location, Location, Location!" We can also use the wise words of a business man in pulse - first, note the location (see fig. 2). Next note the correct position of the fingers in the taking of the pulse (see fig. 3).

Vata is found at the position closest to the wrist, at a superficial level (the level of a light touch). Pitta is found at the middle position and middle level (firm touch). Kapha is found at the position closest to the shoulder at a profound level (deep touch).

    Secrets of Ayurvedic Massage

Very generally speaking, if you find these pulses in other places it indicates vakruti, not prakruti.

Next prakruti is determined by the speed; vata is fast, pitta is medium; and kapha is slow. Now relate this to location. Vata is fast and superficial. Pitta is medium and at a middle level. Kapha is slow and deep.

Now feel the 'quality'. This refers to a subjective view of how the pulse actually moves under your fingers. This is traditionally compared to animals. As most of us do not know how a swan moves it is hard to use these analogies. Think of it as waves on the ocean - vata will be choppy, irregular in size and breadth, quick and erratic. Pitta will be a normal ocean with strong, mid-sized waves that are constant and even in high and breadth.

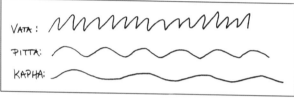

Fig. 4

Kapha will be a calm ocean with slow, deep waves that are equal, low, and farther apart (see fig. 4). To feel the quality it is most important to have a calm mind.

Lastly, feel which part of the tip of your finger that the pulse is hitting. Is it hitting the tip closest to the hand? Vata. Is it hitting the middle of your finger tip? Pitta. Or is it hitting the area closest to the shoulder? Kapha. This helps very much in figuring out the prakruti of the person and is explained in detail by Dr. Lad. Combine all of the above information together to get an idea of the prakruti of the person.

If there seems to be a difference in location and depth it will indicate the vakruti. If there is a difference in location and the finger tips, then this too indicates vakruti. If there is a difference between the speed and any of the others, position, depth, quality and finger tip area, then this too indicates vakruti.

For example, if I feel a fast (vata) pulse in the first position (vata), but at a deep level it can indicate that vata is not at home and has moved into an aggravated or migratory state. Another example can be that of feeling a pitta type pulse, strong and even, at the last position (kapha). This would indicate that pitta has moved into the kapha areas or systems of the body.

Now compare this information. *This is Ayurveda.* Is the prakruti the same as the vakruti? In other words, are the locations, speeds, qualities, and depths consistent? If they are not then they indi-

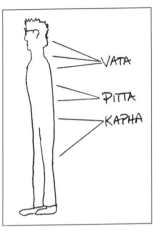

Fig. 5

cate vakruti and also indicate which humor, or humors, is disturbed. Using the first example above, vata disturbance, it would indicate that we need to treat or harmonize vata in the massage that we are going to give. This would influence the kind of massage, the touch used, the oil used, the herbs in the oil, and frequency of the treatments needed to best help the client.

Using the second example, pitta disturbance, it would indicate that we need to treat pitta first and then vata. As all massage works primarily on the prana, or vata humor, it is always considered in the treatment.

In this case it is a secondary consideration. First, treat the vakruti, then the prakruti, and lastly the vata dosha. Usually, the natal nature will be the one that imbalances, i.e., a pitta person will tend to have excess pitta. So treating the pitta in this example will also treat the prakruti or natal nature. This form of treatment in massage is different than other therapeutic methods in Ayurveda where the prakruti is treated first - unless in critical or emergency situations. In massage therapy it is very effective to control the vakruti by first focusing on it and then concentrating on the prakruti as part of the whole treatment.

Don't get worried about the complexity of this. Just begin to do it and after some time it will make sense to you. It is ultimately necessary to study with a teacher to learn pulse diagnosis on a profound level - especially in a more medical sense. For massage this is enough information. If you can distinguish this much it will change how you work with people. Start by trying to understand the prakruti, natal constitution, of the client. Just touching the person in this way, i.e., pulse, will give a more professional feel to your clients. There is no need to tell them you are learning. We are all learning all the time, like the saint in the beginning of the chapter.

The pulse also indicates the upper and lower areas of the body and can show physical problems. The vata point shows the upper

40   *Secrets of Ayurvedic Massage*

body and can indicate the upper back, upper spine, neck and head. The pitta point can indicate the middle of the body and the middle spine. The kapha point shows the lower body and legs (see fig. 5). This is another system than the one I use so I am not well versed in it. The practitioners from Maharishi Mahesh Yogi (TM) often use this system.

Tongue

The tongue is the easiest way to read imbalances (vakruti) in the body. It should always be used in conjunction with pulse, looking at the body, and questioning. The tongue is a map of the three doshas, the internal organs, the body in general, and the prakruti of a person. Reading the tongue is a very refined and exact science. However, you can use simple information immediately in your practice.

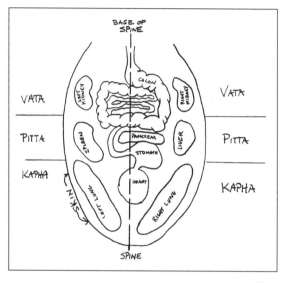

Fig. 6

The size and breadth of the tongue indicates the prakruti of the client. Large, wide tongues are kapha in nature; narrow, thin and unsteady (quivering) tongues are vata; and pitta tongues are in-between as average sized. The back area of the tongue is vata, the middle pitta, and the front kapha (see fig.6). First, look at these locations (remember dad's advise?). What do you see? Look in the mirror now. Come on! Get up and go look. What does the back look like? Rough? Any bumps or tiny pimples? What color is it? Pinkish (normal)? Darkish (high vata)? Is there a film over the tongue? If so, how thick? Two inches (sorry, I have a vivid imagination!)? What color is the film? Repeat this for the middle area, pitta, and the front area, kapha (see fig. 7).

This is useful information concerning the tongue. Colors: vata is a dark tongue and dark in covering; pitta is a red tongue and

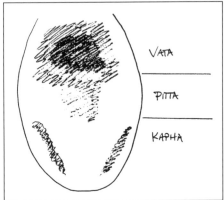

Fig. 7

greenish or yellowish as a covering; Kapha is a pale tongue and white as a covering. Texture: vata is rough and can give tiny pimples, vata can appear as chronic troubles in depressions or mounds; pitta is shiny, as in bright red areas or patches, and cold sores; kapha will have a mucusy texture and appear as pale areas.

Using this information you can see that, for example, if a tongue has bright red tip but a pale overall color, set in a wide large tongue, that the person is probably kapha in prakruti and has an imbalance (vakruti) of pitta in the upper body or chest cavity. Another example can be, a rough middle area of the tongue, set on an average size tongue. This could indicate a vata disturbance in a pitta person. Rough (vata) in the middle (pitta region), set in a middle sized tongue (pitta type person).

Deep cracks or lines in the tongue indicate chronic vata conditions and the person should be directed to a qualified general practitioner to receive general guidance on lifestyle and treatment. A main part of treating chronic vata conditions - or any vata condition is massage. Therefore, if you see these kind of deep lines or cracks, your client needs a long series of treatments. This should however, be put into the context of a general, overall Ayurvedic treatment plan.

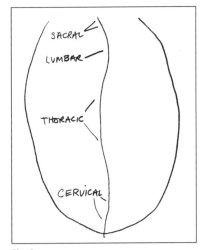

Fig. 8

A deep line, any point, crack, or continuous line on the center of the tongue indicates problems on the spine. These can be physical or emotional. The back of the tongue indicates the base of the spine and the tip is the base of the skull (see fig. 8). Anything on this center line gives you a very good indication of where to

Secrets of Ayurvedic Massage

look for stored emotions or chronic back problems. These lines only appear in chronic cases.

As a rule the tongue is a healthy reddish pink color with a very slight white covering. If there is any major, or extremely strange, condition on the tongue, send them to an Ayurvedic doctor. The same is true for any of the diagnostic methods. Learn what you can do and what your limits are. This is an important part of being a therapist. Develop a group of other professions that you can refer people to if needed.

In summery, a good diagnosis is one that tells you the prakruti of the patient, if there is an imbalance (vakruti), what humor is imbalanced, where in the body the disturbance is located, and what kind of therapeutic approach will be appropriate in relation to the mental state and constitution of the person.

Having this information the massage can begin. How? Read on!

---

[1] Lad, Dr. Vasant, *Secrets of the Pulse*, Albuquerque, NM: The Ayurvedic Institute, 1996

5 Nadis - The Subtle Currents in the Body

"The five senses successively function through the external apparatus, the gross organs, the ears, the skin, the eyes, the tongue and the nose. The senses are subtle; their presence is to be inferred from their functions. They often move outwards."

—Pancadasi, II-7

In Ayurvedic medicine there is a complex, explicit and clear understanding of the human body. It can be summarized as consisting of three doshas (biological humors), seven *Dhatus* (tissue levels), the fourteen *Srotas* (channels - there are 16 for women), and 14 major Nadis (ducts or tubes).

The placement and function of the organs was well understood by ancient Ayurvedic doctors. However, they were given a secondary place to the above mentioned systems. Their perception was that the various channels, gross and subtle, were actually responsible for the health of the individual organs. They viewed the body as an integral unit functioning in harmony and completely interrelated. Thus, the treatment methods in Ayurveda revolve primarily around getting the three doshas in balance and the dhatu, srota and nadi systems to function correctly.

The most subtle of the systems is the nadi system. The other two, the seven tissue levels, dhatus, and the fourteen (or sixteen) channels, srotas, are mostly physical. The seven tissues are the direct result of what we eat. Food is slowly refined throughout the various levels until it ultimately becomes atomic in the form of reproductive fluids. It is atomic in the sense that it is capable of producing life. The channel system carries food, air, blood, waste and primarily physical substances. Although there are channels for the mind and for the prana as well (both of these being different than the nadis).

The prana is the basis of the doshas and the nadis provide a network for them to move throughout the body in their subtle forms and the channels in a gross form. The nadis are the basis of the other two major systems because it is the nadis that circulate the pranas (the five vayus) in the body and that animate the other systems. The nerve tissue (*Majja Dhatu*) and the nerve channel (*Majjavaha Srota*) are fed directly by the vayus in the bone and marrow structure. It is the nadis that transport the vital energy throughout the body. Thus they are the best place for therapy to begin.

Descriptions of the nadis are frequent throughout Vedic and Hindu scriptures. Much of the mythology of India is looked at in a very superficial way, when in fact it is filled with a many deep esoteric meanings. All of the old *Tantric* texts use metaphors to describe the chakras and nadis. This is required to allow only the intelligent, capable student to comprehend the real meaning - thus proving their worth as a disciple and as a recipient of the Divine energy.

One example of this is the story of Lord Krishna and the *gopis* (literally secret, yet also meaning the female cowherds). Krishna was the lover of 16,000 gopis, 200 he was very fond of, and one was his foremost lover, Radha. There are 72,000 nadis in the body, 16,000 which are important, 200 which are primary and one which brings union with god. The Krishna Lila is the dance of the nadis on the awakening of the Self (i.e., Krishna = Self, Gopi = nadi). This is only one example of many.

Yoga scriptures state that there are 72,000 nadis in the body. They are an extremely fine network of subtle channels spread throughout the etheric body (body of prana, pranic sheath, or energetic body). All disease is the result of congestion, blocks or restrictions in the nadi system. Contrary to many occult writers, the pranic body (etheric) permeates the physical. While many people look at the human body as a progression of layers, like an onion, the contrary is actually true. Each body permeates the other to the center of the physical. This then makes it possible for the nadi system to exist in the energetic and physical body simultaneously.

It is not the purpose of this book to go into detail on the nadis and so we will focus mainly on the fourteen major nadis that supply prana to the sense organs, the senses, the organs of action, and the major areas of the body. By using these nadis in massage we can balance the whole pranic function of the body. They relate directly to the five senses and thus the mind. Hence, by working on the nadi system in massage we can achieve a very balanced therapeutic effect on the whole body / mind system. I personally feel this is the primary function of giving massage because all the therapeutic methods in Ayurveda ultimately come down to the treatment of prana. And as the nadis are the channels of the pranas it stands to reason that whatever you do directly on them will be the most effective.

It is possible to work directly on the pranas and nadis without touching the physical body, rather the pranic sheath or body. I worked like this for many years with excellent results. I have outlined this method in *Prana: The Secret of Yogic Healing*. However, it is my experience that pranic healing is best used in the context of the Ayurvedic system where it originated. The information presented here can also be applied to the various "energetic" methods in use today. The efficiency of your work will greatly increase regardless of the therapeutic method you are employing if you understand the nadis and their functions.

Description of the Fourteen Nadis

There are six nadis on the right side and six on the left side of the body. There are two in the middle of the body. This makes fourteen in total. All of these nadis begin from the *Muladhara* chakra, or the root center at the base of the spine.

The body functions in a basic polarity, masculine - feminine, receptive - action, yin - yang, etc. Every tradition has recognized this fundamental polarity in life and in the body. The Vedic sages metaphorically allotted the sun and the moon to represent the active and passive sides of creation. Additionally, they noted that the active side related to the guna rajas and that the passive side related to tamas. The middle channel relates to sattva or to all three gunas as noted by some scholars.

In this sense the use of the gunas is not "negative" meaning that tamas is an undesirable quality to have and rajas only less so as in the case of the mental functioning. The three gunas are part of nature and we would not be able to sleep at night if it were not for the dominance of tamas at night which allows us to sleep. By the same token if it were not for rajas we would not be able to get up in the morning! It is the misplacement of the gunas, or the "wrong" functioning of the gunas that is problematic and eventually causes disease. Hence, when the lunar, feminine nadi *Ida* is referred to as tamasic it is not a judgmental statement. Nor is the reference to the solar, masculine nadi, *Pingala*, a judgment. It is only in the con-

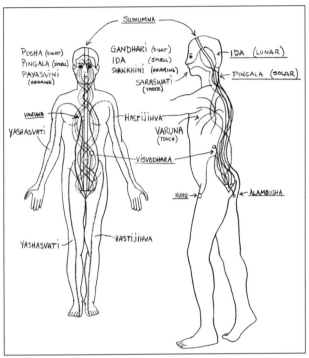

Fig. 9

text of the mind, which is sattvic by nature, that these two gunas are not appropriate.

The Pingala controls and dominates the right side of the body and the Ida controls and dominates the left side of the body. When the prana is moving in one of these nadis all the other nadis associated with it are usually activated as well. The right side is pitta in nature and the left side of the body is kapha in nature. Men in general tend to be slightly more pitta in energy regardless of their prakruti (natal constitution). Women tend to be more kapha in energy regardless of their prakruti. This is due to the functioning of the Pingala and the Ida.

These two nadis intertwine around the central nadi, the *Sushumna*. They cross it four times as they go around the 2nd, 3rd, 4th and 5th chakras (the traditional Yogic locations - *not* the

Western ones). The Sushumna is the most important nadi in the body and goes up - in a metaphoric sense - the center of the spinal column. The six chakras are attached to this nadi and it terminates at the crown of the head or at the *Sahasrapadma* chakra. The crown center is not a chakra in the sense of the other six chakras (see fig. 9).

These are the three main nadis that control all the others in the body. The Sushumna provides the basic energy (prana) for the whole body and uses the chakras to distribute this energy to the various organs and endocrinal glands on a subtle level. It is assisted by the solar and lunar nadis, the Pingala and Ida respectively. All yogic methods, like pranayama and asanas work on these three nadis. Kundalini Yoga works first on the right and left nadis and then on the central nadi by developing and refining the udana vayu - this is supposed to result in the activation of the *Prana Shakti*, or primordial pranic energy. This is supported by a balanced state of ojas and tejas in the body and mind. It is the union of the tejas and ojas that activates the Kundalini energy (Prana Shakti). It then rises to the crown of the head. This 'shakti' must then return from the crown center to the spiritual heart for God (Self) Realization to result. There is reputedly a special nadi for just this purpose, the Brahmi nadi.

It is not the intent of this book to go into the ideas and philosophy of Kundalini Yoga. However, I mention it mostly because there is so much mis-understanding about the phenomenon. Many people will swear that they have experienced the "Kundalini". While it is a common experience to feel the udana prana rushing up and down the spine this is not what is meant by the Prana Shakti or Kundalini. Even a partial awakening of Kundalini will result in supernatural powers or psychological disturbances. In practicing energetic medicine for over twelve years I have yet to met any of the first category, but have met many of the second!

Kundalini Yoga is a method of worshipping the formless in the form of the Divine Mother. If this is not constituting the core of your practice (or of those you know who say they are doing "Kundalini yoga") then there is either a misunderstanding or deception. Dr. Frawley's book, *Tantric Yoga*,[1] gives a good perception of the "right hand" path of Tantric Kundalini Yoga and Dr.

Svoboda's trilogy[2] gives a correct view of the "left hand" path of this Yoga.

Ultimately, how much we, as bodyworkers, can help a person through working on the nadis is insignificant compared to the work the person can do themselves. All natural healing comes back to this point - self responsibility. Any meditation or pranayama practice that a person does will benefit them far more in the long run than a series of bodywork sessions. Hence, it is important that we encourage people to do some form of self work. Bodywork plays an important role in aiding people to begin a right lifestyle or to clear problems that may arise due to outside situations, or past bad habits. Massage therapy in Ayurveda, like all Ayurvedic therapies, must eventually teach the client to practice daily regimes that prevent disease in the first place.

Central Nadis

1. Sushumna - runs from the base of the spine to the crown. Provides the general upward movement of pure prana that nourishes the whole body.
2. Alambusha - runs from the beginning of the Sushumna to the anus. Provides the outlet for impure prana to leave the body.

Right Nadis

3. Kuhu - runs from the base of the spine up to the second chakra and then goes to the end of the penis or vagina. Provides prana to the reproductive and urinary tracts.
4. Varuna - runs from the base of the spine up to the fourth chakra and then branches out to provide prana all over the whole body. It is said to exist everywhere.
5. Yashasvati - runs from the base of the spine to the third chakra at the navel and then branches out to the right arm and the right leg. Provides prana to the limbs and allows movement.
6. Pusha - runs from the base of the spine to the sixth chakra at the 'third eye' and then branches out to provide prana to the right eye.

7. Payasvini - runs from the base of the spine to the sixth chakra at the 'third eye' and then branches out to provide prana to the right ear.
8. Pingala - runs from the base of the spine to the sixth chakra at the 'third eye' and then branches out to provide prana to the right nasal passage.

Left Nadis

9. Visvodhara - runs from the base of the spine to the third chakra at the navel and then branches out to provide prana to the stomach area.
10. Hastijihva - runs from the base of the spine to the third chakra at the navel and then branches out to the left arm and the left leg. Provides prana to the limbs and allows movement.
11. Saraswati - runs from the base of the spine to the fifth chakra at the throat and then branches out to provide prana to the tongue and mouth.
12. Gandhari - runs from the base of the spine to the sixth chakra at the 'third eye' and then branches out to provide prana to the left eye.
13. Shankhini - runs from the base of the spine to the sixth chakra at the 'third eye' and then branches out to provide prana to the left ear.
14. Ida - runs from the base of the spine to the sixth chakra at the 'third eye' and then branches out to provide prana to the left nasal passage.

By looking at these nadis we can see that eight of them come in pairs. The Ida and Pingala serve to bring prana in and out from the nasal and sinus passages and control the sense of smell. The Shankhini and the Payasvini control the ears and the sense of hearing. The Gandhari and the Pusha control the eyes and the sense of sight. The Hastijihva and the Yashasvati control the motor actions of the limbs and thus movement.

The remaining six control the other motor actions or senses. The Saraswati controls taste and the tongue. Visvodhara controls the digestive system and the ability to digest. Kuhu controls the reproductive and urinary systems. And Varuna controls respiration, circulation, the skin and thus the sense of touch. The Alambusha controls the action of elimination and the Sushumna controls the nervous system and the whole body, it contains all other nadis as it is the central pillar of the subtle body (etheric, astral and mental bodies in the Western system).

How to Treat the Nadis

The primary use of the nadis in Ayurvedic massage is to pacify the motor functions and the five senses. Both of these are controlled by the vata dosha (vayu). The classic Ayurvedic texts state that vata is responsible for most diseases. By treating the nadi system we have a direct means to pacify vata. *This is one of the most important applications of massage therapy in Ayurveda.*

This form of massage is called *Abhyanga*, which generally falls under the classification of general massage. Abhyanga also means the massage that we can do daily as part of our Ayurvedic regime. Abhyanga can also mean massage as a preventive therapeutic method, i.e., one that balances or pacifies the three doshas. Consciously using the nadis in massage you can achieve both a method of pacifying vata (including the senses and motor functions) and of disease prevention.

The other form of massage therapy in Ayurveda falls under the category of *Snehana*. Snehana is properly part of Pancha Karma and is primarily concerned with the application of oil and not massage technique as mentioned in the introduction. Although it is possible to work on the nadis in Snehana, it is not really the correct place. Snehana is a whole process of which applying oil massage is but a part. Hence, treatment of the nadis falls under the classification of Abhyanga.

Treatments

1. Sushumna - Apply warm oil to the crown of the head with light clockwise circular motions. (Brahmi oil)
2. Alambusha - It is not appropriate to treat this nadi on others. For self treatment wash daily and apply sesame oil.
3. Kuhu - It is not appropriate to treat this nadi on others. For self treatment wash daily and apply sesame oil.

4. Varuna - All massage techniques treat this nadi. Oil massage is the most effective to treat the skin as an organ of touch. The amount and kind of oil depends on the constitution (prakruti).

5. Yashasvati - Apply warm oil to the palms of the hands and the soles of the feet daily. Use oil according to your prakruti.

6. Pusha - Soak a cotton pad in *triphala ghee,* or in a triphala decoction, or in chamomile tea and then place this wet - slightly dripping - pad on the eyes while you do the rest of the massage. Or apply a little oil and slight pressure to the points above the eye - on the eyebrow.

7. Payasvini - Use an eye dropper to put two drops of oil into the ear (Brahmi or sesame oil). Or put oil on your finger tip and gently apply this oil in the ear. Massaging the whole ear also helps.

8. Pingala - Use an eye dropper to put two drops of oil into the nostril (Brahmi or sesame oil). Or apply a little oil and light pressure one the side of the nostril.

9. Visvodhara - Apply a warm oil massage to the abdomen area. Use oil according to the prakruti of the person.

10. Hastijihva - Apply warm oil to the palms of the hands and the soles of the feet daily. Use oil according to the prakruti.

11. Saraswati - Apply a little oil to the throat and jaw area. A light massage on the sides of the throat and jaw muscles works to treat this nadi. Also, massage the back of the neck. For self care you should clean your tongue daily.

12. Gandhari - Same as Pusha.

13. Shankhini - Same as Payasvini.

14. Ida - Same as Pingala.

One of the most important methods of treating the nadis is through our own daily maintenance routines. This is primarily concerned with proper hygiene and the correct use of the senses. An overloading of the senses is one of the main causes of diseases. Massage therapy is very effective in combating the abuse or overloading of the senses. Nevertheless, this treatment should begin with ourselves. We, as healthcare practitioners, must be aware how we use not only our mind but the other sense organs as well. The importance of this is often overlooked or underestimated. *Do not make this error!*

The sense organs, including the subtle sense qualities of the mind, are the key to long term health. The over use of these organs is the cause of disturbing vata and the whole body - this results in disease. Ultimately, it is the misuse of the senses that, coupled with out of control desires, creates vasanas and samskaras (stored impressions, see Chapter Three).

These latent impressions are directly responsible for ignorance. By this it is meant ignorance on all levels. Starting with the mundane level of the physical body -i.e., ignorance is the cause of diseases - up to the ignorance of our true undying nature. Hence, the control and proper maintenance of the sense organs and the senses - thus the nadis and pranas - is paramount for our health, physically, mentally and spiritually.

Ayurvedic health regimes are very strong on this kind of maintenance. It is advisable to first integrate these methods into your own life and then introduce them to your clients. The basics are: daily cleaning, proper stimulation - not excessive - and nourishment. Oil massage is one of the most important methods of nourishment in daily Ayurvedic health regimes. Cold pressed, naturally extracted oils are extremely high in vitamins, minerals and nutrients. The skin, as you have now learned, is an organ of assimilation and relates to the sense of touch. Oil nourishes the whole body through the Varuna nadi system (the Varuna nadi is actually a very complex system of minute canals that exist over the whole body).

A key factor of self care is the maintenance of the nostrils. As the two nostrils are the outlet for the Ida and Pingala (and these two being the support of all other nadis) they are the most direct and important place of treatment in the body. The daily cleansing and nourishment of the nasal passages has always held a high place in Ayurvedic and yogic health regimes. Now you know why. After cleansing, which is done with the head tilted back and sideways, allowing a stream of warm salted water to pass through, the nasal passages can be nourished with oil. Drops can be put directly into the nose. If this is done daily then the brain is nourished and the vata dosha is held in balance. A simple eye dropper and small glass bottle with sesame oil is a very convenient way to directly work on containing vata when you travel - apply three or four drops on each side before and after travel.

Other forms of nourishment are silence, being in nature, love, wholesome food in moderate quantities, and meditation. The highest form of nourishment is to not think. To disassociate from the perpetual stream of individual thoughts that is called thinking. This then allows your true nature to emerge, dispelling ignorance and bringing happiness and health. This can be done by meditating on the prana and the consciousness that is inherent within.

> "I contemplate that infinite consciousness which is the indwelling presence in the prana but which is neither with prana not other than prana. I contemplate that consciousness which is the prana of prana, which is the life of life, which alone is responsible for the preservation of the body; which is the mind of mind; the intelligence in the intellect; the reality in the ego sense. I salute the consciousness which is the source for both prana and apana, which is the energy in both prana and apana and which enables the senses to function."[3]

[1] Frawley, Dr. David, *Tantric Yoga and the Wisdom Goddesses*, Salt Lake City, UT: Passage Press, 1994

[2] Svoboda, Dr. Robert, *Aghora: At the Left Hand of God*, Albuquerque, NM: Brotherhood of Life Publishing, 1986

_____, *Aghora II: Kundalini*, Albuquerque, NM: Brotherhood of Life Publishing, 1993

_____, *Aghora III: The Law of Karma*, Albuquerque, NM: Brotherhood of Life Publishing, 1997

[3] *Yoga Vasistha*, *"The Supreme Yoga"* Vols. I & II, Swami Venkatesananda trans., Shivanandanagar, Uttar Pradesh, India: Divine Life Society, 1991, Vol. I, page 370

6 Marmas - The Subtle Pressure Points in the Body

*"The pranas which pervade the body and give power
and motion to the eyes and other senses constitute the
vital sheath. It is not the Self because it is devoid
of consciousness."*

—Pancadasi, III-5

According to legend there is a tree near mount Meru that is never destroyed in each cycle of time. When the Lord Shiva begins the dance of destruction as Nataraj the seven worlds are destroyed and everything within them is also destroyed. Each new cycle starts when the Lord of creation, Brahma, sings the song of creation. That is, everything is destroyed at the end of each time cycle except for this one tree and its occupant, Bushunda the Crow.

Bushunda and his tree retreat into their subtle bodies (of which the astral body is a part) and exist there until the world is formed again. Bushunda has lived an infinite number of time cycles in this way and is the wisest being alive. It was Bushunda who taught the immortal Vedic seer Vasistha the science of prana - of immortality. By mastering the prana all powers are achieved and immortality results. It is by knowing and understanding the movement of prana in the nadis that the prana is mastered. The door into the nadis is threefold: through the mind, breathing (prana) and through the marmas. Bushunda says this:

*"Enclosed right in the middle of this body are the subtle ida
and pingala. There are three lotus-like wheels. These wheels*

57

*are composed of bones and flesh. When the vital air wets the
wheels, the petals or the radii of the these lotus-like wheels
begins to vibrate. The vital airs expand on account of their
expansion. These nadis thereupon radiate above and below.
Sages call these vital airs by different names - prana, apana,
samana, udana, and vyana, on account of their diverse
functions. These functions derive their energy from the central
psychic center which is the heart-lotus.*

*"That energy which thus vibrates in the heart-lotus is known as
prana: it enables the eye to see, the skin to feel, the mouth to
speak, the food to be digested and it performs all the functions
of the body. It has two different roles, one above and one
below, and it is then known as prana and apana respectively.
I am devoted to them, which are free from fatigue, which shine
like the sun and moon in the heart...."[1]*

This is a classic description in yoga of a marma. Marma means
secret, hidden. Marmas are points on the body that can give life
and death. The marmas are anatomical places on the body, mostly
composed of flesh and bones. They are an integral part of
Ayurveda and they offer a direct means to treat the nadis and the
prana within them. The three ancient texts that form the three
pillars of Ayurveda, the *Caraka Samhita*, the *Sushruta Samhita*,
and the *Astanga Hrdayam*, all talk about the marma points. The
text by Sushruta deals with them extensively as it is primarily
concerned with surgery. Knowledge of the marmas was mandatory for a surgeon, yet all physicians knew of them and the threat
to life that they hold should they be injured.

Marmas are similar to the pressure points used in reflexology
and acupressure. In fact, it is the system of marmas that is the
origin of these systems and acupuncture. Their use in the context of the Ayurvedic system greatly enhances their results. A
very good reference to the historical origins and nature of acupuncture in Ayurveda is presented by Dr. Ros in his book.[2] Like
acupuncture, the marmas are measured by finger units. There
are 107 marma points and the Astanga Hrdayam further divides
them in to six divisions:

Secrets of Ayurvedic Massage

"Marma is that place which has unusual throbbing and pain on touch. The marmas (vital spots) are so called because they cause death; and they are the meeting place of muscle, bones, tendons, arteries, veins, and joints, life entirely resides in them (any injury or assault to these cause danger to life). They are indicated by the predominant structure found in them; on this basis the marmas are of six kinds. They are one kind only on the common factor, "as seats of life." "[3]

The six divisions that Vagbhata, the author of the Astanga Hrdayam, refers to are as follows:

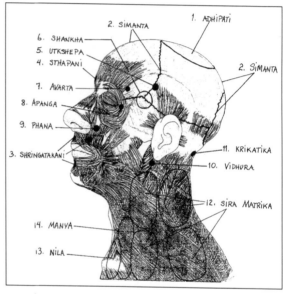

1. Mamsa marmas - are a predominance of muscle tissue

2. Asthi marmas - have a predominance of bone

3. Snayu marmas - have a predominance of tendons and ligaments

4. Dhamani marmas - are a predominance of arteries

5. Sira marmas - are a predominance of veins

6. Sandhi marmas - have a predominance of bony joints

Fig. 10

The marmas are further defined by their location and number on the body:

1. Head and Neck   37
2. Front of the Body   12
3. Upper Limbs   22
4. Back of the Body   14
5. Lower Limbs   22

   Total   107 *(see figs. 10, 11, 12 & 13)*

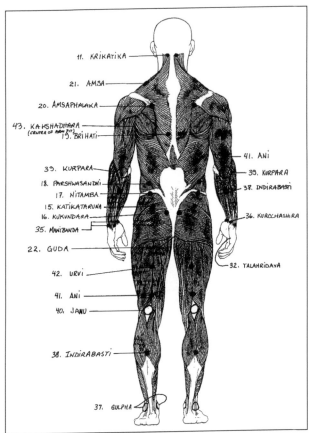

11. KRIKATIKA
21. AMSA
20. AMSAPHALAKA
43. KAKSHADHARA (CENTER OF ARM PIT)
13. BRIHATI
41. ANI
39. KURPARA
39. KURPARA
18. PARSHWASANDHI
38. INDIRABASTI
17. NITAMBA
15. KATIKATARUNA
16. KUKUNDARA
36. KURCCHASHIRA
35. MANIBANDA
22. GUDA
32. TALAHRIDAYA
42. URVI
41. ANI
40. JANU
38. INDIRABASTI
37. GULPHA

Fig. 11

They are also described by the signs they show when injured. I have not included this information as it is more medical in nature. In fact this is the major content of information on the marmas in the ancient texts. In their medical sense they are extremely important for accidents, injuries and wounds. As this constitutes the majority of information in the Ayurvedic texts a practitioner who specializes in the treatment of sports injuries and accidents would be well to further research this subject in the texts mentioned above. It is, however, beyond the scope of this book.

There follows a chart that explains the therapeutic use of the marmas. It is helpful to memorize the main marma points. Nonetheless, I personally found that I already knew many of the marmas because of my previous experience of bodywork. The marma points need not be seen as a complicated and difficult system like acupuncture points. They are naturally sensitive points that you probably already know from your experience of working as a masseuse. This was my experience.

If you are at all sensitive you will have discovered the presence of many of these points. However, it is the *therapeutic* utilization that must be learned from Ayurveda. Start by using the ones that you know of already and learn their names, functions and uses from the Ayurvedic standpoint. In this way it is easy,

Secrets of Ayurvedic Massage

and fun, to find that a certain point that you knew of for some time has a different therapeutic function than you thought.

As stated earlier marmas are measured by finger units, *Anguli*. This means the width of the finger *of the patient*. Not your own finger. Many of the locations of marmas are given in this way because each person is made differently and has a different size and proportion. Marmas also differ as compared to other systems in that they vary from one to eight finger widths - often indicating a region of the body and not a point.

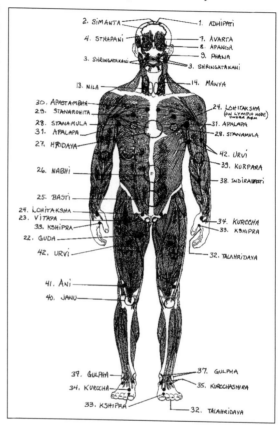

In massage therapy we can use the marmas in three ways:

1. to treat the nadis and thus the pranas
2. to treat a specific organ or system of the body
3. to treat a specific dosha imbalance

Fig. 12

The order and numbering of the marmas is my own system that I use when teaching this information. The order is reversed somewhat from the tradition. Most of the following information on the marmas comes from my teacher Dr. David Frawley and from Dr. Subhash Ranade. The correlation to the five vayus is mostly my own. I find this system of naming the marmas, their locations, and descriptions to be the most accurate. There are other systems, most notably that of South India and Sri Lanka. The South India model has a difference of terminology rather than of its actual nature. The Sri Lanka model may be different due to the strong Buddhist influence, as reflected in all forms of Ayurveda coming from there.

Tables of Marma Points

Head and Neck (*Please note that sizes are given in anguli, or finger widths.*)

N°	Name & Size	Qty.	Location	Composition	Treatment Use
1	Adhipati 4 anguli	1	top of head	joint in Skull	control of mind, nerves & prana vayu
2	Simanta goes linear	5	on joints of skull bones	joint in Skull	control of nerves & prana vayu
3	Shring-atakani 1/2 anguli	4	soft palate	blood	control of nerves & prana vayu
4	Sthapani 1/2 anguli	1	between eyebrows	blood vessels	control of mind, nerves, endocrine glands & prana vayu
5	Utkshepa 1/2 anguli	2	above Shankha	ligament	control of large intestine & apana vayu
6	Shankha 2 anguli	2	temple between ear & Apanga	bone	control of the large intestine & apana vayu
7	Avarta 1/2 anguli	2	above eyebrows on the sides	joint	controls vision, alochaka pitta, & prana vayu
8	Apanga 1/2 anguli	2	corners of the eyes	blood vessels	controls vision, alochaka pitta, & prana vayu
9	Phana 1/2 anguli	2	both sides of the nostrils	blood vessels	controls the sinus & prana vayu
10	Vidhura 1/2 anguli	2	below both ears	tendon	controls hearing, balance prana vayu
11	Krikatika 1/2 anguli	2	junction of head & neck	joint	releases neck & shoulder tension & udana vayu
12	Sira Matrika 4 anguli	8	4 arteries on each side of the neck	arteries	circulation of the blood to the head and heart, vyana vayu
13	Nila 4 anguli	2	on each side of the larynx	blood vessel	circulation, hoarse voice, udana vayu
14	Manya 4 anguli	2	back of Nila	blood vessel	control of blood circulation, vyana vayu

N°	Name	Qty.	Location	Composition	Treatment Use
15	Katikataruna 1/2 anguli	2	buttocks on center of hip	bone	control of adipose tissue, vyana vayu
16	Kukundara 1/2 anguli	2	next to sacrum, posterior superior Iliac spine	joint	control of second (sex) chakra, apana vayu
17	Nitamba 1/2 anguli	2	4 anguli above and across from the Kukundara	bone	controls kidneys, apana vayu
18	Parsh-wasandhi 1/2 anguli	2	2 anguli above Nitamba	blood vessel	controls adrenal & endocrine glands, prana & samana vayu
19	Brihati 1/2 anguli	2	between the 7th & 8th thoracic vertebra	blood vessel	controls third chakra, samana vayu
20	Amsaph-alaka 1/2 anguli	2	on shoulder blades above Brihati	bone	control of fourth chakra, prana & vyana vayu
21	Amsa 1/2 anguli	2	4 anguli above Amsaphalaka, between shoulder & neck	ligament	control of the fifth chakra, udana vayu

N°	Name	Qty.	Location	Composition	Treatment Use
22	Guda 4 anguli	1	around anus	muscular	control of first chakra, reproductive, urinary, menstrual systems & apana vayu
23	Vitapa 1 anguli	2	2 anguli below Lohitaksha, at the root of the scrotum	muscle and ligaments	treats impotence, fertility, hernia, constipation, menstrual problems & apana vayu
24	Lohitaksha 1/2 anguli	4	joint of groin or shoulders on lymph nodes	blood vessels	treats lymphatic system, circulation & vyana vayu
25	Basti 4 anguli	1	top of pubic bone	ligament	control of kapha & vyana vayu
26	Nabhi 4 anguli	1	around navel	ligament	control of small intestine, pachaka pitta & samana vayu
27	Hridaya 4 anguli	1	middle of sternum	blood vessel	control of sadhaka pitta & vyana vayu
28	Stanamula 2 anguli	2	just below the nipples	blood vessels	treats heart, high / low blood pressure, circulation, sadhaka pitta & vyana vayu
29	Stana-rohita 1/2 anguli	2	2 anguli above Stanamula	muscular	treats the breasts, increases milk production, prana & vyana vayu
30	Apasta-mbha 1/2 anguli	2	between the nipples and collar bone	blood vessels	treats lung problems & vyana vayu
31	Apalapa 1/2 anguli	2	lateral side of the Stanamula	blood vessels	controls blood circulation to arms & vyana vayu

N°	Name	Qty.	Location	Composition	Treatment Use
32	Talahridaya 1/2 anguli	4	in the center of both the palms and the soles	muscular	stimulating the lungs, heart to some degree & vyana vayu
33	Kshipra 1/2 anguli	4	between thumb & index finger - & the first & second toes	tendons	stimulation of the heart, prana & vyana vayu
34	Kurccha 1 anguli	4	2 anguli above Kshipra, root of thumb or 1st toe	tendon	foot controls Alochaka Pitta, hand controls prana vayu
35	Mani-banda 1 anguli	4	Just below wrist joint, or in front of the ankle joint	tendon	stimulation of the stomach, pachaka pitta & samana vayu
36	Kurcch-ashira 2 anguli	2	on wrist joint	joint	treats wrist, stimulates nerves & vyana vayu
37	Gulpha 2 anguli	2	on ankle joint	joint	treats ankles, sciatica, arthritis & vyana vayu
38	Indirabasti 1/2 anguli	4	in the mid-forearm & mid-calf regions	muscular	stimulation of Agni, sm. intestine, pachaka pitta & samana vayu
39	Kurpara 3 anguli	2	on elbow	joint	stimulation of liver, spleen & ranjaka pitta & samana vayu
40	Janu 3 anguli	2	on knee	joint	stimulation of liver, spleen & ranjaka pitta & samana vayu
41	Ani 1/2 anguli	4	on the arms and legs 3 anguli above Kurpara & Janu	tendon	stimulation of kidneys & apana vayu
42	Urvi 1 anguli	4	in the middle of the upper arm or thigh	blood vessels	stimulation of the water metabolism, vyana & apana vayu
43	Kaksh-adhara 1 anguli	2	2 anguli above Lohitaksha in shoulder joint	ligament	treats shoulders & vyana vayu

Treatment Methods

The marmas are primarily treated with pressure, circular massage, oil, and essential oils. They can be treated with heat also. They are very delicate points on the body and should not be approached forcefully or aggressively. Likewise pressure should be applied slowly and increasingly stronger. Your mental presence is of utmost importance. Your breathing is critical in all techniques of massage, but most important when you work on the marmas as they are direct doors to the prana of the patient.

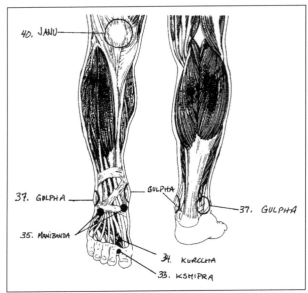

Fig. 13

40. JANU

37. GULPHA

35. MANIBANDA

GULPHA

37. GULPHA

34. KURCCHA

33. KSHIPRA

Breathing

Breathing is the prime method to treat the marmas so it is given first. Breath is the main vehicle that prana uses to enter the body. By the conscious use of breath we can increase the amount of prana that we are projecting to our client. In spite of you or anything you do this is happening anyway. Thus, an intelligent person will utilize the natural functions of nature to increase the effectiveness of their work.

Prana comes in the body on the inhalation (prana vayu) and leaves the body on the exhalation (apana vayu). This polarity is happening all the time. Additionally, the nadi that is dominant at the time of the session will also influence the nature of prana projected, lunar or solar. When prana is consciously projected it can take on the qualities of the other pranas rather than just remaining as apana vayu. This is accomplished by "becoming" the quality that you wish to project versus "thinking" about it.

Secrets of Ayurvedic Massage

For example if you wish to project a hot prana to stimulate and activate the marma you would "feel" the quality of samana vayu which is fire in nature. One way to do this is to "feel" hot yourself or imagine yourself to be in the center of a flame.

Another example of this is to use a cooling calming prana to harmonize a marma, like the vyana vayu. This is accomplished by "feeling" the unity that the vyana vayu provides. Vyana binds, holds and harmonizes. It is cool and feminine in nature. "Feel" the coolness of water as it binds and holds together, as if you are sitting in a quiet pond of cool water. Imagine this as you breath in and out.

This can also be accomplished by controlling the nostril that you breath in from. If you have such a good control over your inhalation then you can inhale through the left nostril to collect and give lunar, cool prana and inhale through the right nostril to collect and give hot, solar prana.

All exhalation should be done out through the mouth. This is due to the active nature of giving. Exhalation through the nose will not give as much prana to the client as the nadis are closed. This form of breathing, nasal, is appropriate for meditation, asanas, or any activity that you do for yourself. If you speak to someone your mouth is open. The same in communicating prana. The Hastijihva and Yashasvati nadis open at the palms to give more prana when the mouth is open on the exhalation. People who talk a lot get drained of their energy in this manner.

Follow the steps in exercise two in Chapter Three to learn how to breath correctly to transmit prana. There is only one difference - that of the exhalation through the mouth. By breathing in this manner you will not deplete your own prana; you will give a higher quality of health promoting prana (prana and vyana vayus); and you will remain mentally present in your work. It does require some practice, but is not really difficult if you have some experience in hatha yoga or meditation. For more information on using prana consciously in sessions refer to *Prana: The Secret of Yogic Healing*.

As you touch the marma point and either apply pressure or massage exhale with the conscious awareness that prana is leaving your hands or fingers. This simple addition will increase the therapeutic effect of your massage tremendously. For more experienced practitioners they can then regulate the *quality* of the prana to meet the needs of the patient. This means the stimulating, calming, penetrating, dispersing, binding or other actions needed to treat the marma. This should be done at all stages of the massage, but especially while working on the marmas.

Pressure

Pressure is used on the marmas in the same manner as any other kind of pressure therapy. The marma is first found and located by the practitioner finding a painful, hard, tender, or sensitive point. Then he / she applies an increasing amount of pressure. Conscious breathing is important and one should exhale with the knowledge that prana is going out of your fingers and into the marma. When enough pressure has been applied that persons feels discomfort you may choose to use small counter clockwise motions to break up the tension of the point.

In general clockwise movements give and stimulate a marma (or the body) and a counter clockwise movement liberates and dispels blocked or stagnant prana. Some practitioners use only clockwise movements. There is nothing wrong in this approach and the results are still good. I prefer to work in a precise manner (as you may have noticed by now!) and use, whenever possible, the natural functions of nature. The clockwise and anticlockwise movement on the body is one such example.

The key to using pressure therapy on a marma is to go slowly until the patient feels discomfort and then go a little more - slowly. I often prefer to just apply pressure alone without any movements. I find that on very hard tense places I apply pressure and hold for about 2 - 3 minutes and then relax for two complete breathing cycles (my own) and once more apply pressure. I repeat this as many times as necessary to liberate the marma. If you consciously give prana you will find that the point clears in half the normal time. If after three times of doing this the point is not much better I leave it alone for ten minutes and then return. I can repeat this several times as well.

With any of the methods in this book force of any kind is not only detrimental, it is forbidden. Force - i.e., pushing through tissues or marmas *because you think it is good* - is a blatant form of violence. There is a very real need for deep tissue work and forceful hard massage. This is not what I am talking about. I am making an important distinction between allowing the body to naturally liberate its tensions and pain versus the practitioner forcing the process. Any experienced and sensitive bodyworker will be aware of this already and of the damage that it can do to the patient / practitioner relationship and the healing process of the client.

Violent, forceful practices on the part of the bodyworker are also self damaging. This indicates a lack of internal harmony and self awareness. The result of this professionally is an accumulation of the patients karma's - especially their disease karma's. If you are falling sick a lot or are depressed a lot when you work with people then you should closely examine how you work with people. The bottom line is that it is your ego that is forcing. Love and ego do not exist together. If there is force, there is no love. There is no stronger healing force in the universe than love. The use of the ego in the session not only forces your will on the person, it also blocks you from receiving love, perhaps even out of the professional context.

Circular Massage

As stated before there are two types of circular movements - clockwise and anti-clockwise. Clockwise circles are for charging, energizing and stimulating deficient or "low energy" marmas. Anti-clockwise movements are to break up stagnant or blocked energy in a marma. Consciously projecting prana during massage is very important as it increases the effectiveness of the massage action.

The method that I prefer is to find the point, locate its center and begin fast, light, anti-clockwise movements spiraling out to the periphery. Then, once at the perimeter, or outer limit of the marma, I change to fast, light clockwise movements back in towards the center. This process can be done several times. Three times is a good number. I use this as a general treatment for all marmas.

For a deficient marma - I guess you've been wondering what the difference between a deficient and stagnated marma is! This does require some further explanation, doesn't it? Deficient means lacking the ability to absorb prana, or losing prana. Stagnant means the marma is neither bringing in nor throwing out prana, its stuck.

This can be felt in the following way:

Deficient feels lose, painful superficially, sensitive, yielding, cold, the surrounding area is cool and lose feeling, muscle tone is lacking.

Stagnant feels hard, pain on a deep level, sensitive with deep pressure, firm, stiff, hot or warm, the surrounding area is tender.

Essentially, both types will need to be charged or energized. However, it is more efficient if the stagnant marmas are "opened and cleansed" before energizing. Hence, it is better with blocked or stuck points to apply vigorous anti-clockwise movements for several minutes before attempting to stimulate with clockwise motions. The contrary is also true, it is better to stimulate a deficient marma with only clockwise movements for several minutes. All motions should be in varying pressure depending on the need, and fast or vigorous. Stagnated marmas need deeper pressure than deficient marmas. Be alert to take into account the location of the body with this information. A marma on the head will not except as much pressure as on the leg or arm as the bone structure will prohibit deep penetration.

Oil and Essential Oils

Oil will be covered in a separate chapter so I will only cover its use briefly here. Essential oils are more concentrated and often stronger for the treatments of marmas as a separate form of treatment - i.e., you have a headache and want to relieve it. In this kind of symptomatic treatment essential oils are the best form of oil to use. They are more concentrated and often - but not always - have a deeper penetrating power. I find them very effective in local application or in the above mentioned example.

I use essential oils to add into massage oils and this is the primary application that I use them for. This is, of course, a personal preference. It by no means indicates a limit of the therapeutic action of these kind of oils. I can refer you to several good books in this regard. The classic book of Melanie Sachs[4] and the innovative book of the Drs. Light and Bryan Miller[5] are good references in this regard. I encourage anyone interested in using essential oils to do so on the marmas as it will increase the effectiveness of the treatment.

Oil is a kind of wonder drug. The modern Western prophet, occultist and healer Edgar Cayce used hot compresses of castor oil to treat a huge variety of diseases and ailments - quite successfully I might add. This kind of treatment has been known for thousands of years in Ayurveda.

Oil in regard to the marmas should first be utilized according to the therapeutic need, i.e., prakruti, dosha, system (srota), and then organ, in that order. If you are treating a specific ailment then this can be added after the dosha. Oil should always be hot or at least warm. This opens the pores of the skin and allows the oil to be more easily absorbed. Oil should be applied with the massage techniques outlined above as they will allow the oil to penetrate deeper into the marma. Oil is beneficial to nourish the nadis and marmas. It is a form of strengthening the body and falls under fortification therapies.

Consequently, if the client is weak or very sickly then oil treatment of the marmas is recommended. Warm oil can be applied, or poured on to a point and allowed to sit for some time before massaging it into the marma. I find this quite effective sometimes as it helps to loosen and relax the patient before actual massage of the marma begins. Again the oil should be massaged in with increasingly vigorous circular motions. Oil massage should also be applied with the conscious projection of prana as it helps to enrich the oil and opens the marma to receive more oil and healing energy.

[1] *Yoga Vasistha*, *"The Supreme Yoga"* Vols. I & II, Swami Venkatesananda trans., Shivanandanagar, Uttar Pradesh, India: Divine Life Society, 1991, Vol. I, pg. 367

[2] Ros, Dr. Frank, *The Lost Secrets of Ayurvedic Acupuncture*, Twin Lakes, WI: Lotus Press, 1994

[3] *Astanga Hrdayam*, vols.; I - III, trans. Murthy, Prof. K.R. Srikantha, Varanasi, India; Krishnadas Academy, 3rd ed. 1996 pgs. 427 -8 Vol. I

[4] Sachs, Melanie, *Ayurvedic Beauty Care*, Lotus Press, WI: Twin Lakes, 1994

[5] Miller, Dr. Light & Dr. Bryan, *Ayurveda & Aromatherapy*, Twin Lakes, WI: Lotus Press, 1995

7 Different Kinds of Touch

"Non-attachment, forgiveness, generosity are products of sattva. Desire, anger, avarice, effort are produced by rajas. Lethargy, confusion, drowsiness are reproduced by tamas. When sattva functions in the mind, merit is acquired; when rajas functions, demerit is produced; when tamas functions, neither merit nor demerit is produced, but life is wasted for nothing."
—Pancadasi, II-13-16

When you touch a person you are sending a clear communication in a not so very subtle manner. How have you been communicating to others through your touch? When you touch another person your 'being' - with the help of prana - goes into the other person.

How we communicate depends on who we are, how much 'work' we have done on ourselves. Hence the importance of meditation and the spiritual orientation of Ayurveda. By this I am not implying that you need to follow Hindu philosophy or religion. I mean that you should first understand what is happening both energetically and mentally, and second, that you are a peaceful, loving person. The result of all types of spiritual practices is to bring a greater awareness of our nature and its interrelationship with the cosmos. The result of this should be internal peace and a loving nature (if it isn't, then it may be wise to question deeply the method, practice or path that you are using).

The Vedic system of knowledge offers a very precise, complete system that encompasses the physical, mental, subtle, and spiritual manifestations of reality. There is no other system that offers such a comprehensive view of reality. In fact the Vedic (as being different from Hindu, which came much later) system is and always has been simply an observation of the cosmic laws of nature. Within this context I will attempt to explain the art of communicating by touch.

A student asked his teacher: "Can you physically prove that reality is an illusion?" The teacher responded thus:

"Concepts cannot be proven and that is what illusions and reality are. Illusions and reality (i.e., *Maya*) do not exist, as the river doesn't exist in a mirage. The truth cannot be proven or experienced. Everybody is involved in this illusion, but they don't know who she is. Learn from Kabir to be happy and eternally in bliss. He sings to Maya: *You are a great deceiver, nobody recognizes you. But I know who you are.*"

The source of touch is this eternal bliss that mystics, like Kabir, abide in. One should first look within to find the source of touch. Its source is the same source as the mind, or the mental process. Behind the individual "I" or sense of personality (ego, but not limited to the Freudian sense) there is a deep sense of being; called *Ahamkar* in Sanskrit.

From the Ahamkar arises the three individualized gunas that we have spoken about several times in this book, and which are a key factor in Ayurveda. Sattva (harmony, peace) is the nature of the 'mind' - as described here - and the senses. Tamas (inertia, latent) is the source of the five states of matter, called the Five Elements by modern writers. Rajas (action, agitation) and sattva and tamas arise from this deep, profound sense of being that we can only know in a state of profound insight or meditation. This is often called 'beingness'.

Sattva creates three groups of functions: the five senses, the five motor organs and the 'mind'. The mind has already been described as including the intellect, emotions, memory, reasoning, feelings, sub-conscious, basic intelligence, and a conscious field of awareness. The five motor organs have also been introduced in the section on the nadis, Chapter Five. They consist of the mouth (to speak), the hands (to touch), the feet (to walk, move), the reproductive organs (to create life), and the anus (to eliminate). These correspond to the five senses of hearing (ears), feeling (skin), seeing (eyes), tasting (tongue), and smelling (nose). The pranas, through the nadis, control all of these functions.

There is another subtle force (for lack of a better word!) that is described as the actual power of the senses. It is, in fact, the senses in a latent or astral form. The Sanskrit term for these astral or subtle senses is *Tanmatras*. The Tanmatras are actually the source of the senses. *The Tanmatras are the link between the object of perception and the sense organ.* They are also the latent or subtle form of the five states of matter, or the *link* to the five elements. *They are the cause of matter to take form on a subtle level.* I think of them as the "functioning" of the five senses, five actions, and five states of matter. They are another pranic function.

They are the link or source of "feeling" and of "touch". We often talk about the "sense of touch" - this is the tanmatra of touch. By refining our senses we can begin to feel the "sense of the sense" of touch - the tanmatra. This is not mandatory for massage - it is a secret. By finding in yourself the tanmatra of touch a whole new world will open up before you.

I found this almost by accident. I love prana. I was mad about working with prana and spent three to four hours per day in meditation and doing pranic exercise. Additionally, I was working on clients each day - usually two or three. This helped to develop my ability to feel the movement of the prana in my body and in my clients. My mind - and so by association the pranas - became still, or active when needed. I could (can) feel the subtle bodies easily with my hands and the movements and congestion's within them.

However, this is not what enabled me to touch the Tanmatras. Some years later, through the grace of my teacher (not to mention a lot of hard work on his part!), my mental functioning stopped and I fell into the Ahamkar. At that time I perceived the Tanmatras. The mind must be absent for the Tanmatras to reveal themselves. They are too subtle to perceive when there is other activity.

Once I was able to identify them and their activity due to the prana, I was able to sense them in my work sessions. This is a very subtle concept and even more subtle in the context of a massage. Bluntly, it is the most subtle thing in existence because it is before the senses, i.e., before you sense anything. There is a relation here to intuition, yet it is still the tanmatra that allows intuition to function as the "sixth sense". I encourage you to explore this avenue further as it will open a much broader vision to your work. According to the yogic texts *mastering* the Tanmatras - which is not what I am talking about - gives one the control of the five elements and the manifestation.

Remember that in massage you are not touching skin, tissues and ligaments; you are touching a part of the divine. First touch your own inner divinity, then you become qualified to touch that part of the divine in another. This is the true healing power of massage. Massages lacking this divineness lacks love and so the power to heal.

The Three Kinds of Touch in Ayurvedic Massage

In Ayurveda three kinds of touch are recognized. They correspond to the three gunas - sattva, rajas and tamas - and indicate an appropriate therapeutic response to different individuals and their needs. The three forms of touch can be used in both Abhyanga (daily, therapeutic) and Snehana (oleation, oil massage) massage. However, they are more properly defined as belonging to Abhyanga as Snehana is mostly concerned with the application of oil - the oil itself being the therapeutic agent - not the touch per se. Still, the touch should be adjusted to the constitution and condition of the person.

Three kinds of touch exist for the different constitutional types of people (prakruti). Three kinds of touch exist for the different imbalanced states of people (vakruti). Three kinds of touch exist for the psychological state of people (guna predominance and mental prakruti). In this way Ayurveda has a touch or combination of touches that suits all people and their therapeutic needs.

Sattvic Touch

Sattva indicates harmony and a state of flexibility. A sattvic touch is one that is loving, gentle and soft. It is sensitive and intuitive. It increases the guna of sattva in the person. It is relaxing, harmonizing, balancing and rejuvenating emotionally. It effects the mind and thus our feelings and emotions. It nourishes the nerves, nadis and pranas. It is the most peaceful and harmonizing of the touches on the five pranas and so the body. It indicates a refined approach of the mind and technique of the practitioner. It is the best approach to calm the nadis that terminate in the sense organs.

The sattvic touch is best suited for vata people or those with vata vakruti. Mixed prakruti's like vata/pitta and vata/kapha should also be treated with a sattvic touch, at least to begin with. For that matter, it is recommended by many people (and I agree) that every person should be approached with a sattvic touch to begin. This kind of touch is good to calm rajas people and allow them to open to deeper work. Sattvic touch is good for thin or fragile people.

Oil plays an important part in the sattvic touch. The oil provides ample lubrication which facilitates the gentle approach of sattva. Yet, the oil itself, depending on the herbs decocted in it, can be of a high sattvic quality also, such as Shatavari, Ashwagandha, or Brahmi. The oil works as a physical medium to transmit prana from the practitioner to the client. Vegetable oils are generally sattvic in quality and so aid in this form of touch. Oil is used in good amounts for vata people.

A sattvic touch is appropriate for mental or emotion disturbances regardless of the prakruti, again at least to open the person or to create the possibility of an opening. A sattvic touch is good for many things, but is not stimulating or clearing. Hence, it should be used whenever you are unsure what to do or for chronic nervous disorders. The most sattvic of all touches is to not touch the body, but rather to touch the pranic body. This is very effective for many conditions and sensitive people - it is not appropriate for tamasic, or rajasic people.

Rajasic Touch

Rajas indicates a state of change, action and movement. A rajasic touch falls between the light sattvic and deep tamasic touch. It is firm yet not painful, strong yet not rough. It is a touch that seeks movement, it seeks to open and stimulate. It is very effective to work on the first tissue levels (dhatus) plasma, blood and muscles. It is moderate and probing, searching for points or places of congestion. It generally is considered to be good for pitta types or persons with a moderate build.

The rajasic touch is appropriate for work on the marmas. The marmas are best stimulated by this touch. A sattvic touch is generally too light for the marmas unless you know how to impart large amounts of prana directly to the point. The marmas need stimulating and clearing work in order to activate the nadi or nadis that they relate to. A small quantity of oil should be used with the rajasic touch. This helps the general lubrication of the massage and provides nourishment to the skin. Care should be given not to overheat the person with this kind of touch as pitta people are already warm. Enough cooling oil should be used to facilitate this.

A rajasic touch is done firmly and with a steady rhythm this creates heat and change. It is best suited for people in general good health, pitta prakruti, muscular tensions, chronic pains, poor circulation, clogged lymphatic system, poor stamina, and who have sedentary life styles. This kind of touch works through stagnation and opens up the circulation of the plasma, lymph, blood, nerves, and pranic systems.

Tamasic Touch

Tamas indicates a state that is blocked, stuck or held - as in a belief. A tamasic touch is one that opens and liberates. It is deep, strong and penetrating. It can be invasive and painful if done improperly. Pain is not a 'given' in deep tissue work, nor is it mandatory. In Ayurveda this often indicates an improper preparation of the client. In the West many deep tissue practitioners smile and grin with pleasure as they 'break up knots', sending the client out the window with pain (this reflects on the ignorance of the practitioner - not necessarily the method). This will be explained further in Chapter Nine.

Tamasic touch is meant to be used on places or regions where a rajasic touch is ineffective. Often it is needed to un-block or liberate a mass of tension in the body. At this level of deep tissue work it is naive to believe that physical habits or situations are the sole cause of the problem. The nature of tamas, and so the deep levels that it relates to, is one of holding and stagnation. This kind of blockage is directly related to the mind and subtle body - i.e., mental functioning, emotion, feeling and pranic function. If a practitioner try's to do deep tissue work without the proper preparation and explanation to the client then the work is bound to fail or be much less effective.

Tamas indicates a boundary or barrier that is set - mentally or in the body. The tamasic touch is meant to break this barrier. However, as the nature of tamas is not to move one must bring rajas into the mind and energetic system of the person in order to have success. Yoga always uses rajas to move or change tamas, to bring it toward sattva. Ayurveda functions in the same manner. Hence, the correct preparation is necessary for the tamasic touch to be truly effective and not just painful.

This touch is done without oil, or very little, instead it uses dry powders. Its action is rough, aggravating and stimulating. It is appropriate for kapha types of people. The tamasic touch is good for weight control programs, especially as a part of a greater program. It is very effective to stimulate the metabolism and ignite the dhatu agnis (tissue fires, or metabolic function in the tissues - i.e., burn up fat). This touch is good for people with large body's and thick deep skin. It is done with a clear purpose in mind and strongly. If done excessively it can create strong resistance and blocks.

A balanced approach is the best. The touch should be chosen that fits the prakruti of the person, then adjusted to fit the vakruti of the person. A rajasic touch is needed to break and stimulate the muscle tissues. It is often best to use the tamasic and rajasic touches together and to use the sattvic touch to prepare and finish. A tamasic touch is seldom, if ever, appropriate for vata people. The best way to lose a vata client is to use a tamasic touch in your first session.

Practical Exercises

Here are some practical exercises to understand and develop the three kinds of touch. In doing these exercises remember that what you feel or do on a subtle level has a greater impact than what you do on a gross level. For example you can go to a therapist who is good technically vs. one who makes you feel good just to see or talk with. The first has developed the gross or physical skills and the second has developed the subtle, or person. The best is a balanced approach that accounts for both the subtle and the physical. These techniques are to try and help you find the subtle qualities of the touch as the physical side is rather obvious: soft, invigorating and deep.

(Please note: breathing into your throat is not necessarily more sattvic than into your lower abdomen. No location in the body is more sattvic than another, these gunas are much more subtle than that. Each exercise is designed to activate certain latent energies within you and so they use different places and methods of breathing.)

Exercise One

Close your eyes and relax sitting in a chair or on the floor. Breath a few times to relax further. Breath with your nose and into your throat and then down into your lungs with long relaxed breaths. Focus your attention on your heart area as the destination of the inhalation. On the exhalation allow the breath to leave through your hands. Repeat this for ten cycles of breathing, each cycle imagine yourself becoming a little more relaxed and your breath a little longer and deeper.

Now imagine the person that you love and respect the most. This can be someone from the past or present, alive or not. It could be your personal deity, guru, or just a member of your family. Hold their image as you continue with the breathing. Imagine that you are touching that person and that each time you exhale the energy of the heart area is leaving you and entering into their body. Imagine it as an offering, as a gift. Imagine that you are offering your love and that they are accepting it. A flow of inhalation and exhalation. You are inhaling love from the universe and giving it to the person that you most respect and love - as a gift.

This is a sattvic touch, warm, loving, peaceful, harmonizing and gentle.

Exercise Two

Close your eyes and relax sitting in a chair or on the floor. Breath a few times to relax further. Breath into your lower abdomen with normal breaths. Feel the air entering into your nose and then going down to your belly directly. Feel the navel as your destination of the incoming breath. Allow the breath to leave out through your hands. Your breath should not be deep or shallow - just normal. Breath into your belly, navel area, and out through the hands. Repeat ten cycles of breathing like this.

Now imagine that you have a practice, with two nice rooms. A waiting room and a session room. You are working in the session room and you have three people waiting in the office. More people are coming later, you must work fast and very precisely if you are going to get your work done and keep the clients happy. There is no room for mistakes or for spacing out. See how your breathing is now. Is it faster? Keep it regular and normal. Feel the breath enter directly into your navel area. Concentrate on your client, on your work, be precise in your movements. Feel that knot? Work on it, go through it - breath, that's right, keep your breath moving - move that knot. Let your hands go through the knots, keep your breath moving.......

This is a rajasic touch, stimulating, precise, active and moving.

Exercise Three

Close your eyes and relax sitting in a chair or on the floor. Breath a few times to relax further. Now breath into your nose and down to your pelvis area, below the navel. Make this point your destination for the incoming breath, breath down as far as you can. On the exhalation allow the breath to leave out through the hands. Let your breathing be relaxed yet strong, more on the deep side, with a strong emphasis on the exhalation. Breath like this for ten cycles.

Now imagine yourself in a strong storm. The wind is so strong that you have trouble staying on your feet. The rain is pounding you with such force that you can hardly see. There is a flood around you. You are holding your small child in one hand and a fence post in the other. Your breath keeps you rooted to the ground, the deeper you breath down the more you are rooted to the earth. As you exhale the breath grips your child and the post through your hands. Your purpose is clear, if you let go of your child the wind will tear them away and drown him in the flood around you. If you waver your grip on the post it will loosen and you will drown also. You breath deep and with power, the breath flows out and holds you firmly and powerfully to your child and the post. Breath down deep and exhale through the hands.....

This is a tamasic touch, powerful, purposeful and strong.

Remember that the touch of the touch, the sense of the sense is the tanmatra. Look deep within as you become more sensitive and try to find the source of the three touches - the tanmatra of touch. This will give you the best control of touch and enable you to touch the minds and hearts of those you work with.

8 The Appropriate Use of Oils, Herbs and Powders

"The body which is produced from the seed and blood of the parents, which are in turn formed out of the food eaten by the parents, grows by food only. The body is not the Self, for it does not exist either before birth or after death."
—Pancadasi, III-3

The skin is an organ of assimilation. What you put on your skin either nourishes or restricts the metabolic function of the body. Nourishing substances build a healthy quality of skin by giving the correct nutrients to the plasma, blood and muscle levels of the body (the 1st, 2nd and 3rd tissue levels, or *Rasa Dhatu, Rakta Dhatu and Mamsa Dhatu*). Restriction happens when an inappropriate substance in put on the skin.

Any substance that is put on the skin is absorbed immediately into the plasma level and then into the blood and muscles. Hence, chemicals or other inorganic substances that are applied to the skin are carried throughout the body by the blood and plasma. They are not confined to the skin alone. When these substances enter into the body there is a disturbance of the metabolism, minor or major depending on the substance and the frequency of application. The long term result of any inorganic substance is to suppress or restrict the metabolic process in the body. This forms toxic material, or *Ama*, in the body.

Ama is generally described as undigested food matter in Ayurveda. Nonetheless, ama is also of a mental nature as well as physical nature. Other physical forms of ama (toxins) are created by the substances we put on our skin and absorb. If the substance is of an organic nature then nourishment and the elimination of toxins results. If it is of an inorganic nature then ama will eventually result, clogging the subtle channels of the skin, plasma, blood and muscles. In all forms of ama the primary question is of *agni*. Agni is generally translated as being the digestive fire. There are, however, agni's at each level of the body. This means that for all seven tissue levels of the body we have an agni, or a principal of digestion, that processes whatever comes to it; organic or inorganic.

The question of agni is paramount in the Ayurvedic system, yes, even in massage. In massage therapy we can increase the agni in the Rasa Dhatu which corresponds to the plasma of the body and the lymphatic system. As plasma is the major component of the body and the lymph system is the primary filter of that component, it stands to reason that the agni - cellular metabolic function - on this level is extremely important for our long term health.

The use of oil is extremely important in the prevention and elimination of ama in the outer layers of the body. The use of creams, lotions and refined oils is not only detrimental, it suppresses the metabolism and increases toxins in the body - reducing your long term health. This may not be apparent immediately, but there is no question that many of the items that people are putting on their skin today is indirectly linked to the cultural weakening of the immune system, among other things. The immune function is weakened by fighting ama and strengthened by the use of nourishing oils that expel ama. Ayurveda states that you should only put things on your skin that you would put in your mouth, i.e., food.

Why are oils so good for the body? Because they are food. In classical Ayurveda all forms of oily products from butter, ghee, vegetable fats, and animal fats were used and classified according to their therapeutic actions. One of these substances stands out as being the best overall product to use generally; sesame oil. Each constitutional type should use the oil that is specific for their constitution. In that context, sesame is the best all around oil for head or foot massage in which it is often recommended regardless of the natal constitution (provided there is no strong imbalance present in which case the vakruti must be addressed).

Vegetable oils contain many vitamins, minerals, enzymes, and prana that strengthen and nourish the body. However, to actually get these qualities from the oil, the oil itself must be 'cold pressed'. This means that the extraction process of getting the oil from the seeds, or whatever, must be done without heat or chemicals. To get this kind of oil one can go to the local health food store. Be careful with manufactured massage oils. If you have an oil that you like, write to the manufacture and ask how the oil is made. *The oil should not come to the boiling point in the manufacturing process.* If it does then the medicinal qualities will be greatly reduced or eliminated.

Oils are useful for massage because they nourish and soothe the skin and muscles. Additionally, when they are absorbed in the body they help to lubricate the lungs and colon, the major sites of vata in the body. Some oils will also nourish the deeper tissue levels of the body, the bones, bone marrow, nerve tissue and the reproductive fluids (see table). Because of this kind of nourishment oil massage can fall under fortification therapies and is very helpful to strengthen weak and convalescing people. Oils are necessary in the body to lubricate the connective tissues and to help in the maintenance of our fat tissue. Oils also provide the lubrication of the various secretions and discharges from the body. For example, constipation is a lack of lubrication in the colon and so many oils are effective in helping elimination of the stool.

Table of the Seven Dhatus or Tissue Levels of the Body

	Dhatu	Sub - Dhatu	Waste Product
1	Plasma & Lymph	-mammary glands and fluids -menstrual flow	mucous
2	Blood (Most specifically Red Blood Cells)	-blood vessels -muscle tendons	digestive bile
3	Muscles	-skin	ear wax, sinus mucous
4	Fat & Connective Tissues	-fatty tissue under skin	sweat
5	Bones	-teeth	nails, body hair
6	Marrow & Nerves	-hair on the head	tears
7	Reproductive Fluids	-ojas	none

If one is using inorganic creams or lotions then you are missing all the possibilities of nourishing your client on a physical level. Meaning that your massage is nourishing their soul, but not their skin and metabolism. These substances are also missing the most fundamental element - the life force, prana. Commercial manufactures have never been able to put the life back into a substance once they have killed it to make the product. There is more consciousness in this area presently with some manufactures, but be very careful when considering to buy a 100% natural product as to the real significance of the word "natural". Boiling is a natural process.

If the right oil is used then there is nothing more effective in nourishing different levels of the body, and if used daily the whole body. Oils can further potentize - increase their potency - by charging them with prana, empowering them with *mantra*, placing them on *yantras*, or by adding herbs. A combination of any of the above is also effective.

With the addition of herbs you not only increase the amount of prana in the oil, you also guide the prana to a specific therapeutic action. This action depends on the base oil and the plant used. In Ayurveda there are classical formulas for each prakruti and for certain common aliments. Additionally, many doctors make their own special oils as do different manufactures in India.

The use of oil is twofold in Ayurvedic massage therapy: first, as a lubricant and as a vehicle for medicinal plants to pacify the three doshas. Second, as part of Snehana, or oleation therapy. The first category falls under daily maintenance routines or Abhyanga. The way that Western therapists practice massage also falls under this category. The second category, Snehana, is both external and internal. The external being massage and the internal being the consumption, or drinking, of oil. This can be used outside of Pancha Karma therapy as was mentioned before.

One example of this is known in South India where certain practitioners are what we would refer to as physical therapists. A specific case that I know of personally involved a young woman in her early thirties. She had a mild scoliosis and some lower back pain. She found a practitioner and he began her on drinking 1/2 cup of oil twice per day for seven days. When this was done he began the deep tissue work and the physical relocation of the bones using enormous amounts of oil externally. She had to lay and sleep at night in a certain position on a flat board. This process went on for two weeks. At the end of this time she was as straight as the board she had been lying on. She then was told to take a three month break and return. During this time she needed to do certain yoga postures and sleep in a special manner. The result was the correction of a condition that modern medicine considers impossible to correct without surgery. She no longer has any pain and she has good posture.

This is not an isolated incident. It is, however, difficult to find a good practitioner in South India as it is anywhere (there, they are not in the yellow pages!). The point is not to run to India, but rather to see the reason why Ayurveda stresses the use of oil therapeutically in massage. Most doctors agree that it requires one day of drinking oil per tissue level (dhatu) of the body, i.e., seven days of drinking oil to penetrate the seven dhatus. This is of course for normal persons and not for special or chronic cases. The internal use of oil lubricates the deep connective tissues and allows deep tissue work to be done more effectively and with little or no pain.

The purpose of all Ayurvedic therapies is to bring peace to the body and mind. When there is peace then the person can properly place their attention on living and pursuing a spiritual life. This is the tradition. Even if a spiritual life is not your goal or goal of your clients, having peace should be. It is hard then in this context to endorse deep tissue work without the proper preparation of the body. Snehana is the system that provides the physical preparation. Chapter Nine will discus the mental preparations necessary for not only successful, but transformative, work.

Use by Constitution

To understand the following information it is helpful to remember the energies of each of the humors. This information is commonly available in introductory books on Ayurveda. I have given a brief description of each dosha so that your memory will be triggered into seeing the relation between the oils, herbs and essentials oils that are beneficial for each constitution

Vata Prakruti

The Vata dosha is cold, dry, fast, irregular, erratic, mobile, light, rough, and dispersing.

The best oils for vata are: sesame, almond, castor, and mustard.

The best herbs to use for vata are: ginger, cinnamon, licorice, ashwagandha, calamus, jatamansi, dashamula ('ten roots'), and valerian.

The best essential oils are: sandalwood, musk, myrrh, and wintergreen.

Notice that the oils, herbs and essential oils that are best for vata are generally opposite in quality. Vata is cold so oils that are warming (see the next section for the energies of oils from the Ayurvedic point of view) will help to pacify vata more than cooler ones. In general all oils are opposite to vata in quality. Hence, oil becomes one of the prime treatment methods for harmonizing the disturbances of vata that we all get from today's society regardless of our constitution.

Sesame oil has an amazing array of vitamins and minerals. Additionally, sesame seeds posses a special enzyme that is very beneficial to the brain. In Ayurveda there is no other oil that is as nutritious as sesame. Each oil has its therapeutic aspect, sesame oils best quality is to nourish the whole body and the mind. It is very sattvic in quality which helps all mental and nervous functions.

Almond oil has anti-oxidant properties and is easily absorbed by the skin. If sesame feels too heavy then use almond oil. This oil is good for people who are unaccustomed to having oil massage and it is still very high in nutrients. Both almond and sesame oils are used in rejuvenation and fortifying therapies. They are contra indicated for toxic states or overly congested persons.

Castor oil is famous for its many uses. Castor oil is very high in certain minerals that build tissue and strengthen the body. It is generally taken internally in the West to help elimination. At the beginning of this century Edgar Cayce used castor oil packs to heal many people from a variety of diseases. His method is direct from Ayurveda, although he had no idea. He used heat to open the pours and stimulate the metabolic function and the oil to drive the toxins from the site into the intestinal system where it could naturally be eliminated. Castor oil is very effective warm to drive out ama from the first tissue levels. It has a special affinity with the female reproductive system and can help premenstrual cramping and pain by applying it locally several times per day externally.

Mustard oil is light and heating, because of this it can be very helpful to use with heavier vata types or dual constitutions that have high vata. It is the oil specifically for kapha types, yet it combats the heaviness that can come from a restriction of vata in the body. Restricted vata is about the same as high kapha. When the five vayus are not moving well then the body becomes heavy and lethargic. This also increases tamas in the mind. Vigorous massage with mustard oil is very effective to stimulate vata and clear the nadis and systems of circulation. In general, vata people should always be massaged with hot oils. They should never be given cold oil at any time. In winter the oil should be hot and in summer one can use warm oils.

In regard to the use of herbs it is best to refer to the *Yoga of Herbs* by Dr. Frawley and Dr. Lad[1] as it is the best source of information for learning the Ayurvedic energies of herbs. Basically, when you mix an herb or plant into the oil the natural qualities of the oil then takes on the quality of the plant. Thus, you have a broader spectrum therapeutic agent than with either one alone.

Take for example the herb Ashwagandha. Ashwagandha is one of the prime herbs for lower vata. It is also one of the prime regenerative herbs in the world. It has the quality to rejuvenate the body and mind, as it is sattvic in quality. To further increase this action one would mix it with sesame oil which is the strongest nutritive oil. To balance this action with that of elimination one would mix it with castor oil and add some ginger and cinnamon to increase the action of driving the toxins out of the tissues, yet strengthening them at the same time. This is often better to do with weak vata types.

It is an art to mix and formulate oils for therapeutic work. One should be trained in herbalism and understand well the Ayurvedic energies of both oils and herbs. As the information on herbs exists already I have given the energetic information on the oils only. This will allow a person to study and formulate their own oils according to the Ayurvedic system.

Essential oils play an important role in massage by nourishing the sense of smell and of the pleasure that they bring to all of the sense organs. I speak about them more specifically in the treatment of marmas. They are very important to add to your massage oils for the fragrance alone. They are also important therapeutically as they are very concentrated oils. They should be used in small amounts - a drop or two - directly on the body or in a dose of 20 drops per 100 ml, or 3 1/2 oz. They are powerful and work strongly on the nadis to stimulate the pranas. They should be treated with respect, especially the stronger oils like wintergreen or eucalyptus.

Pitta Prakruti

The Pitta dosha is hot, oily, mobile, wet, sharp, malodorous, penetrating, and light.

The best oils for pitta are: olive, coconut, sunflower, and ghee.

The best herbs for pitta are: coriander, licorice, turmeric, gotu kola, jatamansi, and shatavari.

The best essential oils for pitta are: sandalwood, rose, lavender, and jasmine.

Once again, notice that the oils, herbs and essential oils for pitta are cooling in nature. Pitta is also oily by nature and so less oil is used externally than with vata. The oils themselves are lighter in quality than for vata too. Olive oil is perhaps the best oil for Westerners to use as it is easily available in a high quality form. If it does not absorb well into the body then try another brand as it probably has been adulterated. Olive oil is also better to use during the day as it has less of a sedative effect than the more nourishing, heavy oils.

Oils should be applied warm in the winter and cool in the summer for pitta types. Attention should be given to the vakruti of the patient before giving cool oils as it can increase ama very quickly. Make sure your client can properly digest the cooler oil before covering their body with it. How? Check their tongue to see if there is a covering of ama already or if the tongue itself has a nice reddish color (the sign of agni).

Coconut is classically listed as the oil of choice for pitta. However, to find a good coconut oil in the United States at a reasonable price is not that easy. It has many good properties and is very good for the skin. It is very high in cholesterol and may not be appropriate for many of your clients. Sunflower is a very good all around oil. It is nutritious and not too heavy. It is the most balanced of the oils in its effects on the three humors. It is very nourishing for the skin and the lymphatic system.

Ghee is not an oil but is clarified butter. This is butter which has been cooked until the solids separate from the liquid. The solids are removed and the golden yellow liquid hardens into a paste. This paste can be used in cooking, as a vehicle to take herbs, or it can be used in massage for pitta people. Ghee is one of the prime rejuvenators in Ayurveda. It has the ability to increase the agni (metabolic fire) in all of the tissue levels without aggravating pitta. It nourishes all seven tissue levels and increases ojas. Ghee can be too heavy for kapha types and for those who are very toxic. In toxic situations it should be combined with ginger, barberry (Berberis vulgaris), and turmeric to aid in burning up the toxins. Ghee may not be appropriate for many of your pitta clients as it has a particular smell and it stays on your skin for some time. Dry powders can be applied over it to remove the excess.

Here again I think going into the individual herbs is beyond the scope of this book and it has already been presented in a better manner than I could by Drs. Frawley and Lad. These two men are leading proponents of Ayurveda in the West and both offer courses in herbalism from time to time. They are worth studying with to have a greater understanding of Ayurveda. Herbs that cool and pacify pitta are given above. Gotu kola (Brahmi) is an outstanding herb to use for pitta. It is very sattvic and not only pacifies pitta it nourishes the brain and nerves. It is my favorite for pitta oils.

The essential oils for pitta are all cooling in nature and should be added to the oil that you use. It will help the therapeutic effect of the oil and the pleasure of having the oil on the body of your client. The scent is very important (especially for the critical minds of pitta!). A therapeutically sound substance that stinks is not going to be well received by anybody.

Kapha Prakruti

The Kapha dosha is cold, wet, slow, stable, dull, heavy, dense, slimy, oily, soft.

The best oils for kapha are: mustard, sunflower, corn, and sesame.

The best herbs for kapha are: cinnamon, ginger, juniper, calamus, dashamula, and bala.

The best essential oils for kapha are: musk, cedar, myrrh, and eucalyptus.

Kapha is usually cold and congested to some extent and so the oils, herbs and essential oils given above are opposite in quality. Kapha needs warm stimulating oils and herbs to get their metabolisms functioning again. The main problem with kapha - generally speaking, mind you - is that their metabolic functions are low. Heating oils and abrasive powders are very useful to correct this tendency.

As mentioned under vata, mustard oil is the oil of choice for kapha as it is light and heating in quality. Sunflower is a good all around oil as mentioned under pitta. And sesame oil is useful when toxic situations are not present. Corn oil is very beneficial for kapha as it is low in cholesterol and can be used when other oils may not work. As kapha is oily by nature very little oil should be used in the Abhyanga methods. The oil itself should be applied hot in winter and warm in summer. Cold oil is never appropriate for kapha types.

Herbs that are heating and stimulating are good for kapha. Herbs are usually used in a powder form on kapha although herbal oils are better than plain oils for kapha. Calamus oil is especially stimulating, nourishing and yet sattvic for kapha types. Essential oils play a more important role for kapha as they are very concentrated forms of oil. They are best applied with vigorous strokes and are very stimulating to the circulation and lymphatic systems.

The Ayurvedic Energies of Oils

Almond Oil - (Prunus amygdalus)

Taste:	sweet, slightly bitter
Attribute:	heavy

Potency:	heating
Long-Term:	sweet
General Action:	good for the kidneys and lungs, nourishes skin and muscle tissues, relieves muscle pain and tension
Specific Action:	demulcent, expectorant, tonic
Therapeutic Action:	lowers vata, increases pitta and kapha

Castor Oil - (Ricinus communis)

Taste:	pungent, sweet, astringent
Attribute:	heavy
Potency:	heating
Long-Term:	pungent
General Action:	digestive stimulant, reduces stiffness in muscles, reduces ama
Specific Action:	demulcent, analgesic, nervine, aphrodisiac, antispasmodic analgesic, helps arthritis, helps complexion and skin, reduces ama and heals sores; warm or hot oil packs reduces swelling, pain and cramps.
Therapeutic Action:	lowers vata, increases pitta

Coconut Oil - (Cocus nucifera)

Taste:	sweet
Attribute:	heavy
Potency:	cooling
Long-Term:	sweet
General Action:	nourishes the lungs and skin
Specific Action:	refrigerant, emollient, tonic, reduces inflammation, psoriasis, eczema, burns, aphrodisiac
Therapeutic Action:	lowers pitta and vata, increases kapha and cholesterol

Corn Oil - (Zea mays)

| Taste: | sweet |
| Attribute: | heavy, drying |

Potency:	cooling
Long-Term:	pungent
General Action:	urinary system, skin
Specific Action:	diuretic, demulcent, alterative, nourishes the skin, very low in cholesterol
Therapeutic Action:	lowers pitta and neutral for kapha, increases vata

Ghee - (Clarified Butter) or Ghrta

Taste:	sweet
Attribute:	heavy
Potency:	cool
Long-Term:	sweet
General Action:	tonic, rejuvenator, aphrodisiac, digestive stimulant, strengthens the liver, kidneys and brain
Specific Action:	tonic, rejuvenator, nourishes all seven dhatus, builds ojas, aids voice and eye-sight; increases all forms of agni
Therapeutic Action:	lowers vata and pitta, mildly increases kapha

Mustard Oil - (Brassica alba)

Taste:	pungent
Attribute:	light
Potency:	heating
Long-Term:	pungent
General Action:	stimulant, relives congestion and heaviness in body
Specific Action:	stimulant, demulcent, expectorant, carminative, anti-fungal and anti-parasitic
Therapeutic Action:	lowers kapha and vata, increases pitta and toxic blood conditions

Olive Oil - (Olea europaea)

Taste:	sweet
Attribute:	light

Potency:	neutral
Long-Term:	sweet
General Action:	nourishes skin and hair
Specific Action:	clears and strengthens liver and gall bladder, laxative, nourishes skin
Therapeutic Action:	lowers vata and pitta, increases kapha

Sesame Oil - (Sesamun indicum)

Taste:	sweet
Attribute:	heavy
Potency:	warming
Long-Term:	sweet
General Action:	nourishes the ears, head, hair, eyes, teeth, bones and female reproductive system, it is a digestive stimulant and tonic.
Specific Action:	nutritive tonic, demulcent, rejuvenator, promotes hair and bone growth
Therapeutic Action:	lowers vata, can aggravate pitta in summer or when pitta is high, also do not use in high ama conditions

Sunflower Oil - (Helianthus annuus)

Taste:	sweet
Attribute:	heavy
Potency:	cool
Long-Term:	sweet
General Action:	strengthens lungs and lymphatic system
Specific Action:	demulcent, helps lungs, treats burns, skin rashes, and sores
Therapeutic Action:	generally balanced, best for pitta and inflammation

Using Herbal Powders in Massage

A word about powders. In Ayurveda when powders are mentioned, it really means *powder*. Not with lumps and bigger bits, but a very uniform sifted powder that is of medicinal quality. It would be very hard to grind up some root or herb yourself and achieve the level of powder that is referred to here. You can do it. But be aware that it involves more than using your coffee grinder. All pieces must be sifted out and ground into powder. The last thing should be to sift the powder to a uniform quality. Many stores that specialize in selling herbs will do this for you. You may also buy these powders easily in the United States (see resource list in the back).

Herbs are used in powder form to provide roughness and abrasive qualities to massage. There is a whole system of qualities or gunas (being different from the three gunas of sattva, rajas and tamas) in Ayurveda. This system give ten pairs of opposites. One must understand this system to understand the use of powders (and oil for that matter). The twenty gunas are as follows:

Heavy	Light
Slow	Fast *(sometimes given as Dull and Sharp)*
Cold	Hot
Oily	Dry
Slimy	Rough
Dense	Liquid
Soft	Hard
Static	Mobile
Subtle	Gross
Cloudy	Clear

Notice that the opposite of slimy is rough. The quality of kapha and pitta - because they both have the water element in them - is oily and sometimes slimy. When the slimy quality is dominant in the body powder is prescribed. Additionally, the opposite of oily is dry. When the skin is too oily then powder is also recommended. As herbs are light in quality powders are also prescribed in cases when a heavy feeling dominates the body. Herbs are also subtle in energy and can be used to combat gross manifestations in the body and mind, such as the lethargy mentally and physically that causes a sedentary life (i.e., couch potato).

One can see that powders are mainly used for kapha, next pitta, and lastly, or rarely, vata. For vata types powders can be used to eliminate the excess oil that remains after giving a massage. Calamus, jatamansi, or valerian can be used if there is excessive nervousness and agitation. Ginger or cinnamon can be used to stimulate and ashwagandha, licorice, dashamula to nourish the body.

Pitta benefits from powder in combination with oil. Pitta people are prone to skin rashes and inflammations. Hence, powders and oils should take this into account. Coconut and sunflower oil are the best oils for skin inflammation and they should be combined with coriander and / or turmeric powders. Turmeric is an exceptionally good herb for all types of skin problems and is fairly close to being tridoshic, or good for all humors. If a skin problem exists it is better to first treat it internally with cold bitter herbs to clean the blood, liver and spleen, all of which are responsible for your skin condition. If there is any strong skin irritation it relates to these organs and the sub-pitta, Bhrajaka. The person should first see an Ayurvedic practitioner to have a dietary and herbal treatment before any kind of external massage work is done. Certain pastes, like turmeric, are good to use externally at the same time, but professional guidance should be sought first. Or you can refer to *Ayurvedic Healing*.[2]

Kapha people are the types most helped by the use of powders in massage therapy. Rough, hard, dry, and light are opposite qualities (gunas) to kapha. By using these qualities in the form of powders and further applied in a deep, vigorous manner one can effectively drive kapha back to its home or pacify it. Powders take a primary role in Abhyanga methods and a secondary or minor role in Snehana therapies.

The herbal powders recommended for kapha are all stimulating and heating. They should be applied in liberal amounts after the light application of the appropriate oil. The point here is to try to drive them into the pores of the skin with deep, firm and vigorous strokes and movements. Kapha people need stimulating massage and deeper pressure to stimulate their metabolisms. Culturally, India is predominately kapha. Because of this, Ayurvedic massage is often perceived as limited to very deep, vigorous and penetrating massage. Most Indians like to have this kind of work, regardless of their constitutions, which is normal for kapha types and their culture.

Some Famous Ayurvedic Oils

Here is a list of some of the more well known oils from Ayurveda. These are simple forms of the recipes. Often these same formulas have thirty different ingredients in them. As most of these ingredients are not available in the West there is little point in referring to them.

Bhringaraj Oil- Bhringaraj and sesame oil
> Good for pitta, balding, premature graying of hair, nourishes the mind

Brahmi Oil - Brahmi (Gotu Kola) and coconut oil (sometimes with sesame oil)
> Good for pitta and vata, nourishes the mind and senses, calms the nerves, improves memory and treats headaches and insomnia.

Calamus Oil - Calamus and sesame oil
> Good for vata, nervous tensions, anxiety, mental disorders

Chandan oil - Chandan (sandalwood) and sesame oil
> Good for pitta, relieves inflammation, burning headaches, and fever

Mahanarayan Oil - Shatavari, Bilva, Ashwagandha, Bala, Castor, Brihati, and sesame oil.
> Good for muscular pain, arthritis, rheumatism and paralysis

Triphala Ghee - Triphala (lit. three fruits, Amalaki, Bibhitaki, Haritaki) and ghee
> While not an oil, it is balancing to all three humors and is good to treat the eyes, head and taken internally to clear ama and increase agni. Externally it is best used on pitta types.

Practice - Making a Herbal Massage Oil

Making a medicated oil is not difficult, but it is time consuming. I have given the method that I use and that is the easiest to do at home. When you do this once or twice you come to appreciate why good medicated oils cost as much as they do.

Start by choosing the formula that you want and buy a high quality of oil and herbs. Do not buy cheap essential oils as they are often adulterated. They last a long time so it is worth it to buy a medicinal quality. When you have all your ingredients together you can begin.

First, make an herbal decoction in water of the herbs you want to use in the combination that you want, i.e., 3 shatavari, 3 ashwagandha, 1 calamus, 1 licorice, and 1 ginger. Put these into warm water at the following ratio of 1/2 ounce of herbs to 1 cup of water. In four cups of water you would then have 2 ounces of herbs, whole, cut or ground. Boil this mixture for one hour and then let stand for an hour. Strain off the herbs and pour the decoction into another pan with an equal amount of oil, i.e., one cup to one cup.

Do not cover the pan. Now cook this mix of oil and decoction over a low heat for about two hours (longer if you are making large amounts, up to eight or nine hours). *Do not bring to a boil.* Cook in this manner until all the water has evaporated and only the oil remains. Check this by dropping a drop of water into the mix, if it cracks then it is ready. Or stir it and see if there is any sign of oil floating on the top of a water like substance. When you are sure that the water has all evaporated then the mix should be allowed to cool. When cool you should bottle it in colored glass bottles. Now in each bottle of oil add twenty-five drops of essential oil to increase the therapeutic action and to harmonize the scent of the mixture. You may mix the essential oils, however, in total they should not exceed thirty drops per 100 ml or 3 1/2 oz of oil. During this process be careful not to burn the oil. Oil by nature is flammable and so care should be taken not to spill it or catch it on fire while processing it. Good luck!

[1] Frawley, Dr. David, & Lad, Dr. Vasant, *The Yoga of Herbs*, Twin Lakes, WI: Lotus Press, 1986

[2] Frawley, Dr. David, *Ayurvedic Healing: A Comprehensive Guide*, Salt Lake City, UT: Passage Press, 1989

9 Three Different Techniques in Massage

"The Self knows all that is knowable. There is no one to know It. It is consciousness or knowledge itself and is different from both the known and the unknown, the knowable and the unknowable."

—Pancadasi, III-18

Many years ago my teacher was staying with some friends and students of his in northwestern India. They very much wanted him to meet a yogi that they knew and tried to convince him for some time. After a few days he gave in to their wishes and the following day the group of five people drove for three hours to the ashram of this yogi.

Now this yogi was special in the sense that he could read minds and give you answers to your questions without you even asking them. Needless to say this attracted quite a crowd on the days that he would see people publicly. He would answer their questions and bless them as was the custom. Now custom also dictates that you give a little, or a lot, of money to the yogi for his blessings. This is the arrangement and everyone seems happy with it.

The five of them arrived and the friends of my teacher, Sri Poonjaji, where quite happy because they thought that the yogi would bless their teacher, adding more merit to their choice of a teacher. They all wrote down their questions on a small piece of paper and put it in their own pocket. Sri Poonjaji went along with it and sat with the many others on the floor until their turn came. The yogi read and answered the questions of everyone in the group, all the while sitting on his platform. Then it was Poonjaji's turn. The yogi looked at him for a moment and then went on to the next person without saying anything.

The friends of my teacher where greatly disappointed. They were rather morose for the rest of the event and when it ended they slowly stood up to leave with everyone else. Then a servant of the yogi came up to Poonjaji and asked him to come to see the yogi in private. The friends were happy again and infinitely curious. It was extremely rare that the yogi saw anyone in private.

Poonjaji went into the yogis room and sat down. The yogi touched his feet and said, "Please teach me the power you have".

Poonjaji replied, "What power are your referring to? I have no powers."

The yogi responded as follows. "I have the power to read the minds of people and to read the papers in their pockets. I spent fifteen years learning this *sidhi* (psychic power). When I came to you, there was nothing in your mind. There was no movement of thought. You have the power of silence. My guru could not teach this to me because he did not have this silence. You are the first man I have met who has this power, please teach it to me."

Poonjaji replied that if he wanted to learn silence then he should abandon his ashram and come with him because he traveled continuously in those days. He never stayed in one place for long. The yogi could not give up his ashram and the lifestyle he had, so he didn't learn what he wanted. My teacher left with his friends much amused. There is no power stronger than silence.

Hence, the foundation of every technique is silence. The stillness of mind is the fundamental element needed for a successful massage. Stillness allows the technique to flow uninhibited from you. It allows you to merge with your client into a deep rapport of beingness. In this state the prana flows effortlessly to your patient. In this state a quality that is not possible to cultivate can arise. This quality some call love, some call it the divine. Whatever the name, this grace can only happen when there is silence. Thinking and love do not exist simultaneously.

Preparation for Massage

Perhaps the most important technique is preparing the patient for the therapy session. This is often overlooked, yet it is fundamental in any therapeutic situation. The failure to properly prepare your client mentally, emotionally and physically will reduce or nullify the effectiveness of your treatment. Proper preparation will enhance or give you dramatically better results using the same technical methods.

The reasons for this are as complicated as the human being and vary from culture to culture. Yet it can be summarized simply: every person is looking for love. Each of us needs to feel cared for and secure before embarking on any kind of therapeutic or transformative process. And as you know, massage can be very transformative. But before this process of transformation can happen the client must feel - at least intuitively - safe and secure. This is the basic environment that you must provide. If this is there then an opening may or may not happen, but at least you have set the stage, or created the possibility for it to happen. This primarily relates to you as a person and your own individual development.

Your work environment is also very important. How you set up your room effects the client and their trust in you. You must choose a personal style that is comfortable for you and keep your space clean and hygienic. You should look, act and be professional - yet relaxed. Your oils and powders should be well kept and professional looking and easy to use. Incense, flowers, and essential oils are all useful to make a good environment for massage. Sometimes props, like soft music, are appropriate therapeutically for certain individuals.

Next there is the physical preparation. This relies on your professional skill to understand the prakruti, the vakruti, the mental prakruti, the overall strength of the client, the age of the client, and their openness to you and your work. Accounting for all these factors may happen in a split second or you may need to talk to the person for five or ten minutes to *realize what the client is capable of receiving.* Failure to correctly understand this can put you in an embarrassing or uncomfortable position. Or you can do what many massage therapists do, throw your own failure back onto the client with remarks like: 'you can't let go', or 'you're holding on', or 'pain is part of the process', or 'those knots sure didn't want to go, but I managed'. These are all examples of how therapists avoid their own responsibility to understand their client and their capability to receive therapy. Therapy is far more effective, especially in the long run, when this is understood.

Ayurveda provides a clear and precise method to 'know your client' that does not exist in other schools of bodywork. While in respect to technique western massage may be more advanced, it is light years behind Ayurveda in using a comprehensive methodology to understand the individuals that they are working with. Many schools do not even recognize individuals at all. These schools want to force the same method on everybody regardless of whether the person can benefit from it or not. This is true ignorance and borders on stupidity. Yet all of these schools and methods are valid and good. It is not the technique in question here, it is the comprehension of your client as an individual that is critical.

How do you feel to be treated as a number in someone's list of people? How do you feel when you are treated as an individual? Wouldn't you want to have therapies personally designed for your body and mind alone? Of course you would. There is not one person alive who does not want individual treatment when possible. Ayurvedic medicine provides this possibility if the practitioner is practicing it according to its true precepts. These precepts are designed to treat individuals with their differences, not people in general.

If you have, or can develop, the ability to understand the natal constitution of the person you are working with you are well on your way to knowing what kind and how much bodywork they will be able to take. When you know the imbalanced state, or vakruti, then you will know what kinds of oils, herbs and techniques to use on the person. This is the Ayurvedic approach to massage and this is why you should learn the basics of diagnosis.

The first preparation is yourself and your mental and pranic state. This is covered in Chapter Three. Next in importance is understanding what your client can take or is ready for. Chapter One gives an explanation of the ten different types of constitutions and covers this. Your clients will fall into these categories generally and guidelines are given to show you what kind of work is usually appropriate for each constitution. Chapter Four covers diagnosis so that you can begin to understand the imbalanced state of your client, or how to keep them balanced. Next in importance is your own prana and its ability to flow into the other. This happens naturally, but can be enhanced by the practices given in Chapter Three.

Next in importance are your therapeutic agents, herbs, oils and essences. These should be applied according to constitution. You can use three basic oils. You do not need six or nine different types of oil to work - although this has its benefits. Three basic oils are all that is needed for you to work with people. Powders are again important and useful, but not totally necessary to work. Essential oils may be the mainstay of your method or they may play a minor role. These will be determined by your own experience, the kind of clients you have, and time.

Last in importance is technique. It is sad but true that many people spend years perfecting techniques and ignoring the other aspects of treating people, starting with themselves. This is one reason why many Western practitioners think that Ayurveda is uninteresting and unsophisticated in its approach to massage. The reality is that Ayurveda is so much more comprehensive that it is overlooked. These people are looking at technique only and not seeing the movie because they are looking at the seat in front of them.

In spite of this misunderstanding there actually are three major techniques in Ayurvedic massage. Additionally, there are many varieties of these three methods. The method I described of working on the marmas also falls under these three basic techniques as do all western methods.

Harmonizing - Sattva

Sattva is harmony. Whatever we do that is harmonizing is sattvic in nature. Hence, any activity or substance that has a harmonious effect is sattvic. Harmonizing massage is indicated when the patient needs to be calmed, pacified, or nourished. This kind of technique is needed when there are nervous disorders, stress, anxiety, hyper-sensitivity, or all forms of vata disturbance.

The harmonizing technique begins with your own harmony. As whatever you are goes directly into the client it is best to begin with five to ten minutes of meditation before working on the patient. When you are centered and calm then begin. If your mind / pranas are disturbed you will not succeed in this method, even though you do the physical movements of the hands correctly.

The basis for the harmonizing technique is shallow, soft, superficial, circular movements of the hands. Clockwise circular movements bring energy into the body and anti clockwise move-

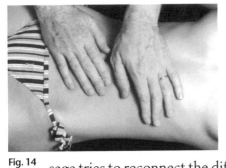

ments liberate trapped energy from the body as I have already described in the chapter on the marmas (see fig.14). The movement can be brisk and energetic, or it can be slow and gentle.

Generally, all of the techniques in Ayurvedic massage are more on the brisk side. This is because mas-

Fig. 14 sage tries to reconnect the different areas and layers of the body. Commonly, only the head is treated with more care, although the scalp and hair are rubbed vigorously when possible. This method is the most gentle and soft of the three. The difference between these three methods is of:

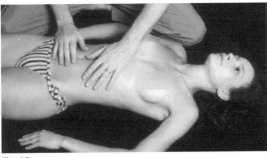

-pressure

-depth

-and movement

As already described the harmonizing method uses circular motions and is most appropriate

Fig. 15

for vata types or vata disturbances in the body. The practitioner should revolve back and forth between clockwise and anti-clockwise circles. This helps to open, liberate and stimulate the plasma, lymphatic system, blood circulation, and nourishes the skin.

The movements should be broad and brisk, covering as much area as is comfortable (see fig. 15). One should begin from the neck and shoulders and work down (see fig. 16). The whole body should be covered in this manner, not only the front and back, but the left and right sides as well.

Harmonizing methods work to calm and harmonize the five pranas. This is especially important on the motor organs or sense organs. This is the correct method to use for pacifying the nadi / pranic / sense function. This is important for overwork, stress, anxiety, and other disorders that abuse the senses. Working on the head harmonizes the prana vayu. Working on the neck and shoulders harmonizes the udana vayu. The heart area calms both the vyana and prana vayus. The navel area calms and harmonizes the samana vayu and below the navel harmonizes the apana vayu. By working on and harmonizing the pranas a deeper level of relaxation is achieved. Remember they control the nervous system.

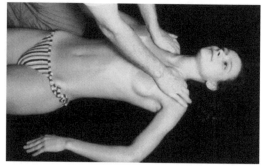
Fig. 16

Sattvic oils are sesame, olive and ghee. These can be used when a harmonizing effect needs to be increased. Flower essences are also very sattvic and can be added to your oils for this purpose. Heating and stimulating oils generally are not used in this general application of harmonizing techniques.

Activating - Rajas

Rajas is action. Whatever we do that is stimulating and activating is rajas in nature. Whatever procedures or products that we use that are stimulating are rajas in quality. Activating massage is for the reconnection of tissues, stimulation of the metabolism, expelling toxins, igniting agni, increasing digestive function, reliving muscular tension, breaking up knots, treating rheumatoid diseases, and arthritis. It is appropriate for all constitutions at times. It is especially good for kapha and pitta people. Vata people should be treated according to their vakruti.

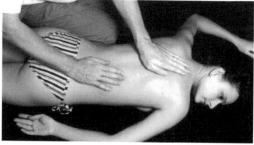
Fig. 17

The activating technique requires the practitioner to be energetic and firm. A silent mind aids this by allowing the pranas to move out freely. The therapist should remain centered and focused on the patient for this method.

The basis for the activating technique is penetrating, firm and brisk movements that vary from a superficial level to a deep level. The strokes are up and down the body (see fig. 17). The hands

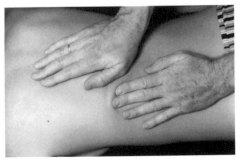
Fig. 18

should be together and rubbing in opposite directions on the superficial level of the skin (see fig. 18). For deeper tissues the strokes should move from top to bottom, from neck towards the feet. All tissues should be pushed downwards and sideways as you follow muscles and tendons downward (see fig. 19). The movements on the superficial level are brisk and fast. On the middle and deep level they are firm and quick.

The activating technique seeks to open and work through hard or closed areas of the body. It does not seek to remove tension

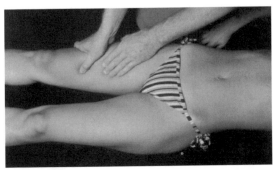
Fig. 19

necessarily. It works to open and move stagnation in the tendons, muscles, nerves, and nadis. One of the primary purposes is (to prepare the ground) for the liberating touch.

The activating method should be done all over the body on a superficial/middle level of tissues before penetrating deeper. The movements should be vigorous and brisk in order to awaken the subtle energies and stimulate the circulation of blood. The increased blood flow will help to dilate the tissues and muscles, thus aiding in deeper work. It should increase the whole metabolic function of the body and reconnect different sites of the body, i.e., lower to upper, calf to thigh. It should be accompanied by enough oil to lubricate the skin, yet also create friction.

With kapha people this is the method and time to use powders. First, apply oil and give a brisk massage to one side of the body, covering the whole body including the sides. Next, apply powder and repeat the same vigorous movements. Be careful to remove all oil from the skin, applying more powder as needed. You should develop a lot of friction and your strokes should be rough and stimulating. When finished repeat on the other side of the body.

Secrets of Ayurvedic Massage

This method works to stimulate the five pranas. General body massage activates the vyana vayu. Working on the neck and shoulders stimulates the udana vayu. Working on the chest and heart area stimulates the prana vayu. Invigorating strokes on the abdomen area stimulates the samana vayu. Working below the navel activates the apana vayu. This technique will stimulate the five pranas and help to liberate toxins and restrictions in the nadis.

Oils and herbs that are heating belong to this method of activating therapy. Oils like castor and mustard are stimulating. It can be appropriate to use cooling oils like olive and coconut with the activating technique. This is primarily true for pitta individuals. There is one prime factor in Ayurveda that must be understood. *Ayurveda is the science of energies.* This means that you can mix any kind of therapeutic approach with any kind of person - provided the energies are understood and the result balances the three humors of vata, pitta and kapha. In other words it may be appropriate to use heating stimulating oils while using a harmonizing technique. Or it may be correct to use cooling, calming oils with vigorous stimulating and activating methods.

Liberating - Tamas

Tamas is inert. Whatever we do that is inert or dull is tamasic in nature. Whatever we do to change stuck or dormant patterns is liberating in quality. It is this liberation of tamasic energies and patterns in the body that we call the liberating technique. To change tamas we need to use rajas. Hence, we need to use the activating touch of rajas to open and create the possibility for the liberation of tamas.

In bodywork we can describe tamas as all the held patterns and habits of the body. In Chapter Three I introduced the Yogic and Ayurvedic understanding of what these patterns and habits are. They are called vasanas and samskaras. These are held in the physical and subtle bodies. Bodywork alone cannot completely liberate these latent impressions. The therapist can assist the client in this process. Yet even here we can only do so on a fairly mundane level - i.e., not touching the main concepts of humanity. This will however result in a very strong and transformative process for the client. Hopefully, this will be the beginning of further internal reflection on the part of the client and supported (again hopefully) by the therapist.

This kind of technique is usually not appropriate on the first session. It may happen naturally on the first session, but that is rare. This work is appropriate for all types of persons in the right situation. It is most appropriate for pitta and kapha. Pure vata types can often achieve the same results through purely energetic methods that touch directly the latent impressions. Such methods like pranic healing and other forms of hands-off work can work very well for vata people if the practitioner is conscious of what is happening. This method can still be useful for vata types, especially those repressed and introverted types.

Impressions are created in this life by the constant repetition of an emotion, feeling, or thought. These not only condition our minds, but also lodge in our tissues throughout the body. Where they go primarily depends on what kind of prana and nadi is involved. Additionally, the situation, like of an accident or strong emotional incident, can dictate the physical location of the impressions. The vasanas and samskaras also tend to collect around different chakras. Which chakra they happen to collect around depends on the psychological / physiological function of that chakra and the nature of the impression. Like will attract like. Still it is the pranas that hold and ultimately liberate the stored impressions. Generally, the impression constricts or restricts the nadi associated with it, causing some kind of pranic disruption. This is why pain or other symptoms are often associated with stored impressions.

By working on the deep tissues we can aid in releasing these impressions. But only if there is the 'space' and energetic affinity with the therapist. By space I mean the psychological space, not the physical space in the body. Really, the release of impressions has little to do with the tissues, other than for them to act as a catalyst in the process. In this respect deep tissue work is a wonderful aid, as many of you know already. Do not, however, confuse the physical tissues with what is really happening.

The best method for releasing these impressions is well known - breath. Yet it is not the breath itself that is doing the job, it is the prana. The standard method taught in the West is to find a place that you feel is holding something, whether it is tension or an emotional impression and slowly go into it with deep pressure - on the patients incoming breath stopping the pressure slightly and on the outgoing breath to apply more pressure. This aids in releasing the tension, etc. What is really going on is that during the out-breath the held tension is becoming liberated by the flowing prana of the therapist. Most therapists will synchronize their own breathing to that of their patients in this kind of deep liberating work - this is correct. Your own out-breath carries most of your prana into the patient, aiding the release of the held prana in the form of tension.

If all the conditions are right - namely that the client has trust in you and is ready to let some held impressions go - then this natural movement of prana will begin to liberate the impressions along with muscular tensions. Consciously developing your own prana is the best aid in this method. Providing a secure and supportive environment is the next most helpful aid. Understanding your clients ability to process and let go of the stored tensions is important. This should be discussed with them over a period of sessions. And you should agree together when deep, penetrating work - that may or may not liberate stored impressions - is appropriate. Even if these samskaras are not touched directly, the whole process will begin to release them over time. Hence, this kind of work is always beneficial, even if nothing special happens in the moment, it will later on.

Here is the method according to the Ayurvedic view. Begin with the activating techniques to open and stimulate the tissues and metabolism in general. Next communicate with your client what you feel is appropriate for them and have them agree to deep liberating work. You can describe it in simple terms - as just tension and pain if appropriate. Or you can describe it as energetic or emotional release. You can describe it as healing traumas or of old wounds. Whatever approach you take it is important that you get approval from your client first. Do not assume that for this kind of work that the fact that they come to you gives you the right to enter into a profound level without their permission. This is all right for the other two methods, but not for this kind of deep work.

When the body is warmed, stimulated and prepared with activating massage and the client is relaxed you may commence. Begin at the upper regions of the body and move downward with your work. This may take several or many sessions to eventually reach the feet. Nevertheless, all these techniques should begin at the neck and end at the feet. The movement is usually from top to bottom.

Go to the first place that you feel tension. Having prepared it already the muscles should be warm and somewhat relaxed, if they are not then stimulate them again with vigorous strokes that are heating and stimulating. Then apply pressure as you breath out, at first with the palm of your hand in a general area. Synchronize your breath with the breath of the client. If the client is not breathing well (shallow or irregular) then bring their attention to your breathing and get them to breath with you. When this is happening apply deep, penetrating pressure with your thumb, fingers, or the knuckles of your first two fingers. Always apply pressure on the exhalation and release it slightly on the inhalation.

The difference between this technique and the previous one is that the other seeks to move through and open. This one seeks to dissolve and liberate the tension through direct confrontation. This technique must be used with the other one. While the other is invigorating this one is penetrating and forceful in its pressure and is unrelenting. Strong steady pressure is required. You must often stay for five or more minutes on one point to dispel and liberate the tension. This is not a quick method. Time, endurance and steady pressure is required. You should not let up the pressure in the area that you are working on until you feel it liberated or the limits of the client have been met.

Much can be done with the palm of the hand before moving to the thumb. The palm is often a better way to release the majority of the tension before using the thumb, fingers, or knuckles to penetrate specific points.

You can accompany this kind of pressure with anti-clockwise circular movements. The purpose of this technique is to penetrate into deep connective tissues or underlying muscles and liberate the tensions held there. This is accomplished mainly with pressure, however, using anti-clockwise circular movements can aid. If it does, use it.

The pressure will cause pain, yet this pain should be able to be released by the patient on the exhalation. If the pain is not released then ease up and move to another location. Never force.

If the body is not willing to release the tension don't force it. Have the client come back for more sessions.

Attention and care should be given to the marma points. Very deep and penetrating techniques are usually not possible or appropriate on the head, neck, chest, and abdomen. These areas are very sensitive and should be massaged with less pressure. Failure to do so can harm the client. Deep pressure is generally OK for the other marma points on the body. Still one should be aware of all marma points and their functions when doing deep tissue work.

10 Abhyanga

"The natural bliss of the Self is uniform and steady, but the mind due to its fickle nature, passes in a moment from joy to sorrow. So both are to be looked upon as the creations of the mind."

—Pancadasi, XIII-74

By now it must be clear that Ayurveda places more emphasis on the practitioner's self knowledge, on understanding the nature of the client, on understanding the imbalance or disease to be treated, on understanding the correct therapeutic agent to use (oil, herbs, etc.), than on actual massage technique.

Technique, however, is important. This is obvious to long time Western practitioners of bodywork. It is not the purpose of this book to ridicule or diminish the importance of technique, rather, prior to this chapter it has been to put technique into its proper place in the Ayurvedic system. It is now our responsibility as Westerners well versed in technique to further enrich the Ayurvedic system with our knowledge - after we have fully embraced the basics that lie within the tradition.

An example of this is obvious in France, where an Indian man has opened "Ayurvedic" schools of massage in France and in Switzerland. His students learn how to massage the hand for a week, the feet for a week, and so on until most parts of the body are covered. His students leave with no comprehension of their own nature much less the patient's prakuti. They are completely unaware of the material covered in the first nine chapters of this book and unfortunately are not able to integrate what techniques they did learn into a complete treatment.

This example is not isolated. It reflects directly on two things: 1.) an approach solely through technique, and 2.) an unqualified teacher. There are other examples in every Western country, not only from Indian nationals claiming to know Ayurveda as if it was a birth right (similar to French nationals claiming to be versed in French cooking or Italians in design), but also from mechanical schools of massage.

The mechanical schools of massage are derived from the allopathic medical tradition (modern medicine). These schools view the body as separate from the mind and emotions - although they will grudgingly, or smirkingly, agree to a psycho-somatic sources of illness. In this school it is thought that the total is made of parts, and if one fails, you fix or replace it. Natural forms of medicine view the body as psycho-somatic and that the mental, emotional and physical states all effect the body as a biological phenomena. This approach feels that you cannot separate the body into parts and address them separately.

Ayurveda goes a step deeper in that it understands the total relationship of the body / mind-emotions / and spirit to the whole universe. This approach is far more general and broad in many respects, yet it can be very precise in its application if needed. Hence, to teach, or learn, Ayurvedic massage without a firsthand knowledge of the profound levels of the inter-relatedness of everything is, in fact, to miss completely Ayurveda.

In order to now integrate all the previous information, I have outlined a basic approach to the main forms of massage in Ayurveda. This is not written in stone, nor will every massage therapist and doctor from the Indian Ayurvedic tradition agree with what I have proposed. To these people I ask leniency and their pardon. I have endeavored to remain true to the Vedic tradition of Ayurveda throughout this book in order to present this amazing system to a broader level of the general population. Therefore, if I veer somewhat here, remember that I am addressing the modern needs of Western society.

In Ayurveda, massage is usually done on the floor, or in some clinics, on a special wooden table that collects and recycles the oils used. Much less oil is used in Abhyanga than in Snehana, as Snehana literally pours on the oil in quantities of quarts at a time. However, some forms of massage can be given on tables, they will be outlined accordingly.

Traditionally, Ayurvedic massage is done in a clinical environment with the doctor overseeing the process. In this context the massage therapists (four therapists are common for one patient) are always of the same sex as the patient. This is for psychological reasons and to prevent the possible disturbance of the patient who has come to be treated. Today it is not always possible for same sex massages. It is, however, advisable. Especially for women practitioners. As our society is obsessed with sex it has made a problem with any and every activity where a person can be abused. Ayurvedic massage is a therapeutic method and if you cannot be 100% professional as a therapist then you have no business being in this field of work - go into sex counseling. Then at least your obsession will be honest.

A note about prana in the actual massage. If your client goes into a controlled, rhythmic breathing - stop them immediately. This is a very common misunderstanding. Controlled or deep rhythmic breathing is just that - control. This is the last thing you want - to have your client controlling anything, much less their own prana. As the prana is the core or root function that the massage is ultimately trying to address, any breath control on the patient's part effectively prevents this. The client should breath normally. For many practitioners of Hatha Yoga this is very difficult. Also for people who do Qi-kong, Tai Chi or other forms of practice that work with breath and 'energy'.

If you see this happening tell them to breath normally. If they refuse or make some kind of comment like 'this is how I always breath' or 'this IS natural', explain to them that any rhythm or control on their part reduces the effectiveness of the massage by 50% and that it prevents you, the practitioner, from really entering into a deep rapport with them and they with you. It provides the possibility to 'let go' of deeper-seated tensions. It is this rapport that will increase the effectiveness by another 50%. If they refuse, honor it, and hope that the next time they will trust a little more, and a little more, until they can breath in a relaxed, normal fashion without control during the treatment.

Their participation with breath in the treatment is appropriate in certain therapies. These kind of situations are outlined below in therapeutic massage. Also, this participation should happen under your guidance, or as it happens naturally, adjust your work to further allow the release through breath.

Outline of a Treatment

"Abhyanga (massage followed by a bath) should be resorted to daily, it wards off old age, exertion and aggravation of vata. It bestows good vision, nourishment to the body, long life, good sleep, good and strong healthy skin. It should be done specifically to the head, ears and feet."[1]

Abhyanga means massage. In general it means daily massage, or the kind of massage that we do on a regular basis to maintain our health. This is primarily what we do in the West. Abhyanga can be divided further into daily massage as preventative maintenance, as a series of therapeutic treatments, or as self massage on a regular basis. I have included self massage techniques in a separate section in Chapter Eleven.

Regular maintenance massage is generally comprised of the harmonizing and activating techniques and uses the sattvic and rajasic touch to work the body. Oil and herbal powders are used according to constitution only and not in great quantities - even for vata types. This form of massage is great daily or bi-weekly as a form of maintenance, especially for the vata dosha and vata people. It relieves muscular tensions and stress. It also nourishes the skin, plasma, lymphatic system, blood circulation, the fat tissues, and the muscles.

Abhyanga as therapeutic massage is somewhat different in that it is targeting an imbalance in the body and working directly to correct it. Therapeutic massage can also be directed towards the release of emotions and other stored impressions that inhibit our lives. In this form of massage it is of paramount importance that the practitioner understands the clients prakruti and vakruti, and that they themselves are in balance and are peaceful. They should have a good understanding of the subtle anatomy and knowledge of the marma points. This form of massage works to balance the three doshas and the five pranas through oils, herbs, the marmas, pacifying the senses, the touch used, and the technique used. It benefits all seven tissue levels and nourishes the whole body / mind / being if done correctly.

General massage guidelines for vata constitutions:

Vata people need light nourishing massage as they are the most sensitive and they their bone structure is the most fragile. Large amounts of oil are very good. The sattvic touch and harmonizing technique are most suited for vata types. But the activating method is very useful to reconnect systems and areas of the body that may have become disconnected. Medicated oils are important for vata. Treatment of the nadis and marmas is enhanced with the use of medicated oils. Pressure on the marmas should always be gentle and harmonizing in nature, pressure can be used when the client is relaxed. Heating oils and herbs are needed. They should be applied warm or hot (not burning). Deep tissue work is rarely advised. If there is any irregularity in bone structure, you are working on a vata person or one with a vata dual constitution; go gently. Massage is especially important at the sites of vata: the colon, pelvis, and chest areas.

General massage guidelines for pitta constitutions:

Pitta people need a mix of a nourishing and liberating kind of massage. They need a mix of sattvic and rajasic touches and techniques. Very fast strokes, like the activating technique, can irritate pitta types if they are over done. They should be started with a harmonizing stroke and then work into a mix of activating and liberating methods. The liberating kind of technique is combined with the activating technique according to the needs they have. Deep tissue work is good for them to release tensions and impression provided they are prepared and notified in advance. Cooling oils and herbs are best for them and the oil should be applied warm in winter or cool in summer. Moderate amounts of oil are used as pitta is already somewhat oily in nature. Do not massage if strong skin inflammations are present unless accompanied by a complete treatment procedure as recommended by an Ayurvedic doctor. For minor inflammations olive and coconut oils are prescribed. Massage is especially important in the abdomen area, the site of pitta.

General massage guidelines for kapha constitutions:

Kapha people need a mix of activating and liberating techniques. They need all three touches, beginning with the sattvic and then working mostly with the rajasic and tamasic touches. Kapha people need a firm approach and must be given strong guidelines and direct instructions. They need warm or hot oils and herbs that stimulate and activate their slow metabolism. They need much less oil, and after oil massage is applied they should be massaged with herbal powders to dry up their skin and to create friction. This further aids in stimulating the body and circulation. Fast vigorous strokes are needed and are the most appropriate for kapha types. Oils are best applied with these fast activating strokes. Deep tissue work is needed from the first massage session onward. It is needed to penetrate the deep levels of tissues and to prevent stagnation in the tissues and systems of the body. Special care should be given to the joints, chest and stomach areas. Vigorous massage in the solar plexus area is very good to ignite agni, the digestive fire.

For all the constitutions it is traditionally said that straight strokes are used on the body and limbs and circular strokes are used on joints. You can apply this to the three techniques outlined in Chapter Nine, allowing for the geography that your hands are passing over.

Practice Exercise for Regular Massage

Begin with yourself. Do one of the meditation methods outlined in Chapter Three. Have your work room clean, warm and professional looking, even if it is for a family member, make a clean space to work in. Next prepare your oils and /or powders, and essential oils. Oils should usually be warm (pitta and kapha) or hot (vata) when you are applying them. Cool oils can be appropriate in summer for pitta people (see Chapter Eight). When you are ready, and your room is ready, then you may begin to work on your client. This method can be done on the floor or on a table.

1. Have your client sit for a moment on the edge of the table or in a chair. Take their pulse or perform the method of diagnosis that you are able to do. Determine their prakruti. Now ask your client to lay down on their back, put a pillow or something under their knees to relieve pressure on the pelvis if needed. Get them comfortable and relaxed. Choose an oil that is correct for the clients constitution (prakruti).

2. Begin with your own breath. Contact your own prana with several breathing cycles and begin with the neck and head. The

neck stores most of our tension and so I always begin with a technique from my first teacher called the 'neck release'. This technique creates space in the body and allows a freedom of movement to the pranas.

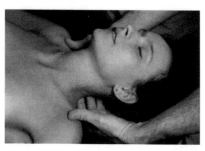

Fig. 20

3. This uses a sattvic touch and only enough oil to moisten your hands, not the client. Place your hands under the neck (C7 - C4) of the patient so that your finger tips align on each side of the spine (see fig. 20). Slowly apply an upward pressure until you have lifted the neck vertebrae about 1/2". Hold this pressure for five of your own breathing cycles. Inhale and feel the prana entering into your body, exhale and feel the prana leaving out through your hands and into

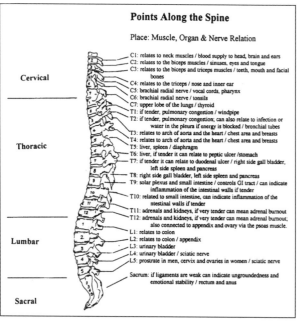

Points Along the Spine

Place: Muscle, Organ & Nerve Relation

Cervical

C1: relates to neck muscles / blood supply to head, brain and ears
C2: relates to the biceps muscles / sinuses, eyes and tongue
C3: relates to the biceps and triceps muscles / teeth, mouth and facial bones
C4: relates to the triceps / nose and inner ear
C5: brachial radial nerve / vocal cords, pharynx
C6: brachial radial nerve / tonsils
C7: upper lobe of the lungs / thyroid

Thoracic

T1: if tender, pulmonary congestion / windpipe
T2: if tender, pulmonary congestion; can also relate to infection or water in the pleura if energy is blocked / bronchial tubes
T3: relates to arch of aorta and the heart / chest area and breasts
T4: relates to arch of aorta and the heart / chest area and breasts
T5: liver, spleen / diaphragm
T6: liver, if tender it can relate to peptic ulcer /stomach
T7: if tender it can relate to duodenal ulcer / right side gall bladder, left side spleen and pancreas
T8: right side gall bladder, left side spleen and pancreas
T9: solar plexus and small intestine / controls GI tract / can indicate inflammation of the intestinal walls if tender
T10: related to small intestine, can indicate inflammation of the ntestinal walls if tender
T11: adrenals and kidneys, if very tender can mean adrenal burnout
T12: adrenals and kidneys, if very tender can mean adrenal burnout; also connected to appendix and ovary via the psoas muscle.

Lumbar

L1: relates to colon
L2: relates to colon / appendix
L3: urinary bladder
L4: urinary bladder / sciatic nerve
L5: prostrate in men, cervix and ovaries in women / sciatic nerve

Sacrum: if ligaments are weak can indicate ungroundedness and emotional stability / rectum and anus

Sacral

Fig. 21

the patient. Now slowly release the pressure and allow the neck to be lowered onto the table, this also takes five breathing cycles. The slower this is done the greater the impression the client has that their neck and head is descending into the table. This treats the Swaraswati nadi and the udana vayu directly.

4. Repeat this again for the upper neck (C4 - C1). Treating the whole neck in this manner treats the nerve endings that control the head and the sense organs residing there (see fig. 21, Chart on the spine /nerve connections).

5. Repeat this again for the head, placing your hands around the

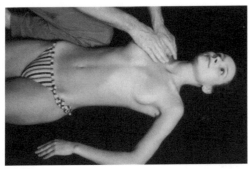
Fig. 22

skull. Your index fingers should be on the base of the skull at the junction of the head and neck or the Krikatika marma (N° 11). Doing this has released much of the superficial tension in the shoulders, neck and head.

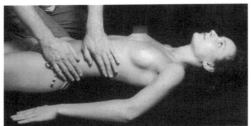
Fig. 23

6. Ask the patient to role over and position them comfortably on the table with a pillow or cushion under the chest and neck, and a pillow or cushion under their shins. They should be comfortable.

7. Apply oil continuously for vata people, for each region of the body for pitta, and only to provide enough lubricated friction for kapha. Begin by using a

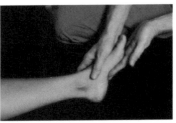
Fig. 25

Fig. 24

sattvic touch and the clockwise harmonizing technique on the shoulders and upper body (see fig. 22). Work your way down each side of the body to the buttocks (see fig. 23). Continue from the buttocks down each leg in clockwise harmonizing movements until both legs have been done (see fig. 24). Do the soles of the feet also (see fig. 25). Apply oil as needed per constitution.

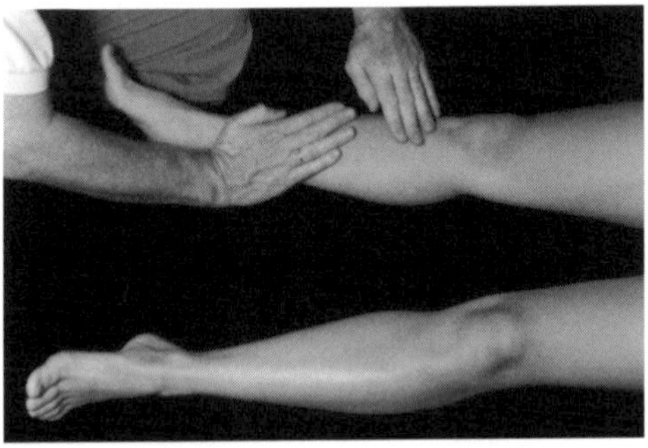

8. For vata people repeat this once more using a combination of anti-clockwise and clockwise movements; use more oil. For pitta and kapha types apply more oil to your hands until they are lu-

Secrets of Ayurvedic Massage

bricated and begin at the shoulders with fast vigorous strokes that activate the body (see fig. 26). These strokes begin on the top of the shoulders and then move down the sides (see fig. 27) and back (see fig. 28). The hands should be side by side and moving in a fast vigorous manner. Do one side of the body down to the feet, then the other side, from shoulders to the feet. For kapha types try to get as much friction as possible. For both types notice areas of tension. For some vata types or mixed vata types you can use the activating method. If the client is very nervous or stressed then wait for another session to use this technique.

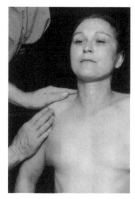

Fig. 26

9. For vata types work on any marma points that may be sensitive, use oil and maintain a sattvic touch. Pressure is also fine to use on the marmas. For pitta types the marma points may need deeper, liberating work, you must feel what is best for the patient, a rajasic touch is appropriate. For kapha the deep liberating technique with the tamasic touch is now appropriate, still be alert that marma points are sensitive. Use a mix of oil and powder - drier than wet - for this work, or use essential oils;

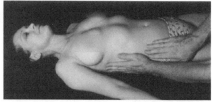

Fig. 27

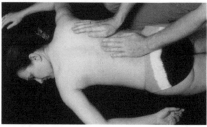

Fig. 28

there should be enough oil to provide lubrication. Move down from the shoulders pinpointing the areas that you found in step 8 that were tension filled. Take as much time as is needed.

10. For all types go slowly down the spine with both hands, one on each side, using oil if needed (see fig. 29). Do this point by point, vertebrae by vertebrae until the sacrum is reached (see fig. 30). If deep tension is felt use the activating or liberating methods and a rajasic or tamasic touch (see fig. 21, Chart of the spine and organ relations). Vata people always need less pressure, careful with their bones as they may have deformations or

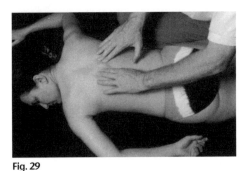

Fig. 29

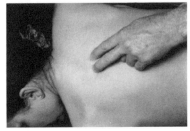

Fig. 30

irregularities, use a rajasic touch to move tension. Now repeat this, starting from the sacrum to the neck (C7).

11. When the back is done, ask the client to roll over onto their back and face the ceiling. Get them comfortable. Take a moment to breath and charge yourself with prana, stretch or do what you need for a moment. Now begin on the front of the body.

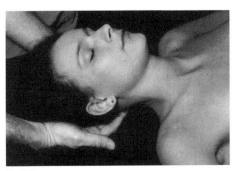

Fig. 31

12. Begin to massage the head at the base of the skull with small circular movements of your fingers. Use a little oil and apply a little pull towards you or to the crown (see fig. 31). Massage the temples and sides of the head, using oil, the harmonizing method, sattvic touch and gently stimulating the marmas - the Utkshepa (N° 5), Shankha (N° 6), Avarta (N° 7), and Apanga (N° 8). Now the face can be done, begin with the forehead. Again gently stimulating the marmas - Simanta (N° 2), Shringatakani (N° 3), Sthapani (N° 4), Phana (N° 9). The neck can be done very softly, avoiding the windpipe and staying mainly on the arteries and ligaments on the sides (see fig. 32). Care should be taken here, or the area should be massaged lightly with oil until a solid client / therapist relation existed. The throat area is very sensitive so watch out before going deeper here. The top of the head should be done last, just apply a little oil on the crown and massage lightly. If your client has a very nice hairstyle you may want to avoid this step and advise them to have their hair done after future sessions.

Secrets of Ayurvedic Massage

13. Begin with harmonizing clockwise circular movements, starting at the shoulders and moving down to the pelvis area (see fig.33). The breasts of women should be massaged gently, even when working on marma points (there are two, one above, and one below the nipples). Move down

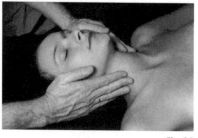

Fig. 32

to the pelvis area, one side at a time. Then do the legs, one at a time, ending on the feet (see fig. 34). *(NOTE: Traditionally, this kind of massage is sometimes given with two therapists working together, one on each side of the body. As this is not practical for Westerners I am describing only the approach of a single therapist doing the work.)*

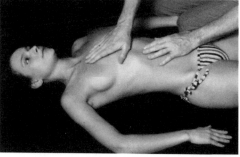

Fig. 33

14. For vata people repeat step 13 once more using a combination of anti-clockwise and clockwise movements; use more oil making sure the

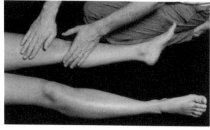

Fig. 34

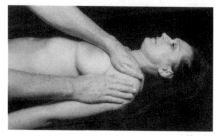

Fig. 35

patient is well oiled. For pitta and kapha types apply more oil to your hands until they are lubricated and begin at the shoulders with fast vigorous strokes that activate the body (see fig. 35). These strokes begin on the top of the shoulders and go down the arm (see fig.36). Then move down the sides (see fig. 37) and then down the front (see fig. 38). The hands should be side by side and moving in a fast vigorous manner. This connects different areas of the body. Do one side of the body down to the feet, then the other side, from shoulders to the feet. Keep pitta types

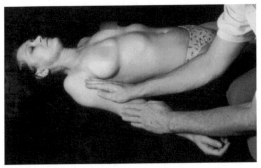
Fig. 36

lubricated. For kapha types try to get as much friction as possible. For both types notice areas of tension. Again, this can also be appropriate for some vata types, use your discretion.

15. For vata types work on any marma points that may be sensitive, use oil and maintain a sattvic touch. For pitta types deeper, liberating work may be suitable on the marmas, you must feel what is best for the patient, a rajasic touch is normally appropriate. For kapha the

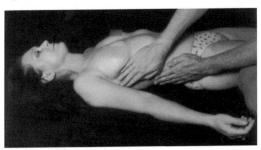
Fig. 37

deep liberating technique with the tamasic touch is now appropriate. Use a mix of oil and powder - drier than wet - for this

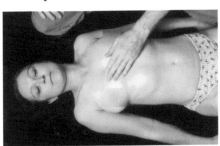

work, or use essential oils; there should be enough oil to provide lubrication. Move down from the shoulders pinpointing the areas that you found in step 14. Do the arms before the side, the sides before the front of the body. Take as much time as is needed.

Fig. 38

16. Apply oil to the main site of the dosha (humor) that is predominate in the constitution; vata- colon, pelvis, lungs; pitta- small intestine, liver and spleen; kapha- stomach, lungs and joints.

17. Now massage the hands well, use the oil suited for the prakruti of the person.

18. Now massage the feet of the person thoroughly, using the oil that is fitting for the prakruti

19. Repeat the neck release to finish the session.

This sequence is generally how I work and it allows room to follow what comes up for the patient and yet covers the techniques presented here. Generally, you can bring the humors down into their 'homes' or sites by warm oil and harmonizing massage (for vata), by cooling oil, a rajasic touch and vigorous strokes (for pitta), and by warming oils, heating herbs, vigorous strokes, liberating methods, and a combination of rajasic and tamasic touches for kapha. This is a very simple, yet effective, way to harmonize the three humors and bring them back to their correct places.

The massage sequence given above falls under strengthening therapies in Ayurveda, or Brimhana. This type of massage is used for strengthening or rejuvenating the patient. It is also used for maintaining the existing health of the person. For already healthy people this is the best form of maintenance.

Practical Exercise for Therapeutic Massage

Start by taking the pulse and using all diagnostic methods available. Determine the natal constitution (prakruti) and the constitution of the moment, or what is covering the natal constitution (vakruti). Compare these two, note the differences. These differences will determine the course of therapies that you are now going to undertake.

Massage as a therapeutic method uses several prime substances (oils and herbs) to work directly on the subtle anatomy. First, this brings the three humors (doshas) into balance, and second, it treats directly any disturbance in the body. Hence, muscle pain will be first treated as a humoral imbalance and secondly as a 'dis-ease'. Disturbances like stress must also include advice from the therapist on how to meditate or otherwise reduce stress before it becomes lodged in the body as pain and tension.

It is in the context of therapeutic massage that the liberating technique is mostly used. In the above description of regular massage the liberating technique can be used. However, once the therapist begins to use this method to change holding patterns it becomes therapeutic and not strengthening, or maintenance orientated, massage.

Additionally, here the marmas and nadis take on an important role in actively treating a disease. For example, if a client comes to you with a history of constipation, you would begin by treating the Shankha (N° 6), Kukundara (N° 16), Brihati (N° 19), Vitapa (N° 23), Kurpara (N° 39) and Janu (N°40) marma points specifically. You would then treat the whole head with nourishing oil and herbs (to pacify the five senses -thus the five pranas) and the lower abdomen with heating oils and herbs (castor or mustard oil, ginger and calamus) to stimulate the colon directly. In this way you can give a massage that is medical in nature, i.e., directly treats an imbalance. This then uses the correct herbs, oils in conjunction with the subtle anatomy, as well as normal tissue oriented massage.

It is really impossible to give all the possible therapeutic methods to use in massage as outlined above. You must learn the idea behind therapeutic massage and not look for a 'cookbook' of treatments. This is not Ayurveda. That approach is a symptomatic way of treating people. Therefore, use the information provided in the earlier chapters as a reference to a clients particular problems. Choose the oils also according to their therapeutic actions as outlined in Chapter Eight. The use of marmas and nadis is a study unto itself in massage, as is the technique of liberating latent impressions. Try the different methods of therapeutic massage and then you will know which suits you the best and concentrate on that method alone until you have mastered it.

For example, the liberation of deep impressions was a strong interest of mine for several years and I worked in such a way to activate these impressions. However, after some time I became more interested in the subtle anatomy and for many years now work more in this direction, that is with marmas and nadis. I do not have all the names of the nadis and marmas memorized myself. Knowing these Sanskrit names is valuable, but I have found that not having the names memorized has not lessened the effect of my work. You must, however, know where they are and what their therapeutic action is.

1. Start with yourself. Become relaxed and focused by using a meditation method.

2. Make a diagnosis and determine what direction your treatment will take. Choose oils and herbs that will suit the clients needs.

3. It is usually best to position the client without pillows or cushions as this type of work is vigorous and they get in the way. Begin with the 'neck release' as outlined above (steps 3 - 5).

4. Have them roll over and follow steps 6 - 7. You may use a cushion under the neck or head here if needed.

5. When the body has been prepared by using the harmonizing technique you can go into a mix of the activating and liberating methods if you feel that (or you have decided in advance with the client) liberating dormant habits and impressions is appropriate. Primarily use the activating method and completely do one side from head to foot, then do the other side; do the arm first before the side of the body. Note the places that are disturbed, tense, or knotted with tension.

6. Now concentrate on using the liberating technique on the points or areas that you have discovered. Follow the guidelines that are explained in Chapter Nine for the liberating method. Breath is very important. Feel your own breath enter your nose and descend to your belly, rise up to your heart area, and rest for a moment. Then let it flow effortlessly out your hands into your client. When you have located and are applying pressure - either with your palm or with your fingers - note the breathing of the client. Use their breath to guide your pressure. If their breathing is not deep enough or even enough to release the pain that is being liberated talk to them and guide their breathing to match yours. This is the right moment to use breath - and so the prana that is actually doing the work - to trigger the release of deep patterns. Nothing special needs to happen here, if it doesn't happen now it will happen later. It also need not be dramatic to be effective as is often recorded in books about therapeutic release. The client should be able to release the majority of the pain and discomfort through their breath. Kapha people can be given this kind of treatment regularly. Very deep work that concentrates only on the connective tissue is more properly placed in Snehana as there is preparation that should be done to the client before proceeding; see the section on Snehana to clarify this point.

7. Alternately, you can work without the liberating technique and concentrate instead on the use of therapeutic oils, herbs,

essential oils, and the marma points. In this kind of therapeutic approach only step six changes, you still prepare the body properly by using steps 1 - 5. Now that the body is prepared you can treat the marmas that correspond to your clients problems. If there is a specific problem then choose the marmas that will help that problem. If the problem is from constriction or restriction of prana then use a more activating stroke. Remember that an anti-clockwise movement releases tension and a clockwise movement charges or give energy to a marma. If the problem is from disruptions of the nervous system or vata, then use the harmonizing strokes. (NOTE: this is quite simple, if the person is very nervous, anxious and generally vata like then use only harmonizing methods; for all other use a more activating circular movement) You should use the oils and herbs that will increase the effectiveness of treating the problem. Like sesame oil and calamus for ungrounded vata types, or olive oil and gotu kola (brahmi) to calm a fiery pitta person, i.e. inflammation of internal tissues. After using activating stokes on the marmas in question finish with using harmonizing movements.

8. You may combine both approaches of liberating and of marmas in the therapeutic massage. This is often the most effective. Do not underestimate the effect of the oils that you use. You should make sure that they are allowed to penetrate well into the skin for vata and pitta types. For kapha allow them to be half in before applying powders to absorb the remaining oils. Pitta may also need powders to remove oils if their skin is already oily. Use the cooling powders like coriander and gotu kola for pitta types.

9. Have the person roll over again and repeat the above methods on the front of the body. Make sure that the client is fairly comfortable. You may lack the time to work on both sides of the body in the same session. I suggest to work the back of the body first in most cases. The exception to this is if the person *has* back problems. In this case work only on the front of the body until a basic flow of pranic energy is once more established. Often by working directly on a problem we further inflame it. In many back problems the client is best prepared by not working on the area in question until the different systems are functioning normally. This can only be determined by you according to each

client. This is specially applicable to vata and pitta types. Kapha types need confrontation usually. The more vata a person is the more important it is to avoid direct confrontation.

10. Take into account that certain areas of the body - like certain chakras - tend to collect certain kinds of patterns or impressions. This is well documented in most schools of massage, such as the inner thighs holding sexual repression, the knees fear, and so on. I personally tend to dislike this kind of classification as it smells of preconceived ideas from the therapist (or the founder of the particular school of massage that they follow). While there is some justification to this it is still best to apply it generally. Ayurveda works on individuals and if you have all these concepts about the body's different parts holding different impressions it does not leave much room for the individual to emerge. I personally do not use any kind of system like this - in other words I am not holding a concept before going into a session. If the client has one of these correspondences happen naturally. Like, 'gee, when you were working on my knees I became afraid', then you can explain that certain types of patterns do tend to collect in certain places of the body. Remember the last time a therapist was working on you and said 'Oh, yea, feel those knots, that's your mother, wow, you sure have all these unresolved issues with your mom'. If you work like this then Ayurvedic massage is not really the right place for you - or you should study deeply the underlying philosophy of Ayurveda to see that these kind of psychological concepts are at best very limited therapeutically and do not touch the deeper healing powers latent in each human being.

11. When the primary therapeutic session is over, i.e., liberating tensions and impressions, or working on the senses and subtle anatomy, you should work on the hands and feet to help further increase the effect of your work. Figure N° 39 shows the nadi correspondence to the organs in the hands and feet. This is important to reinforce your work and also defusing the attention of your client from the deeper work.

12. Finish with the neck release.

This kind of therapeutic massage can fall under the heading

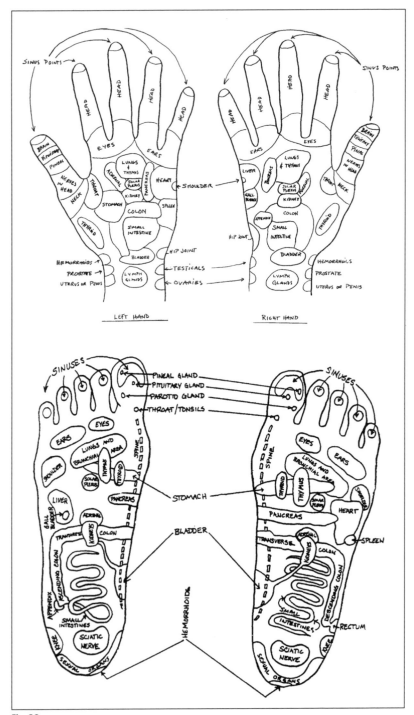

Fig. 39

of reducing therapies (Langhana) in the sense that it activates the metabolism which then burns off excess and so purifies the body. This method, if done regularly and vigorously, can purify the plasma, lymphatic and blood systems which in turn effect the muscle and fat tissue levels. It helps to eliminate excess through its stimulating actions and direct treatment of the marmas, nadis and prana. On the subtle mental level it helps to eliminate trapped or stuck emotional patterns and habits. Most importantly it reduces excess of the three doshas, primarily vata, but the other two as well. Hence, these kind of treatments should eventually be followed by the regular or maintenance type of massage as reducing therapies are always followed by strengthening therapies in Ayurveda.

I should note that there are two primary methods of Abhyanga in Ayurveda; the one I have outlined above (either maintenance or therapeutic) and another. The other school is of the view that all massage strokes should begin from the navel as they believe that the nadis begin from the navel area.

This other school has good points and is worth understanding. By starting all massage strokes from the navel area the basic vitality of the person is harmonized and strengthened. This happens because vata is seated in the pelvis below the navel and is the cause of almost all disease. Furthermore, it is apana vayu which lives in the colon and is responsible for the disease cycle. The sumana vayu that lives in the navel acts as a bridge between the prana and apana vayus and so is important to promote health. Sumana also helps to keep the digestive fire, agni, strong. Having the pelvic / navel area as the main focal point in massage is both strengthening and harmonizing to first vata and then apana vayu. This prevents disease and maintains health. However, it should be pointed out that most yogis consider the chakra at the base of the spine to be the starting point for all of the nadis - not the navel or pelvic area (see chapter 5).

In my own experience of working with clients and teaching I favor the method outlined in this chapter for the following reason. Modern man is centered in the head by the over use and emphasis of the intellect (buddhi) and senses. It is my opinion that Western people benefit more from bringing prana (i.e., the five vayus) down to the pelvic center and feet than by bringing more energy up from the navel to the head area which is the case if you start from the navel. This relaxes the mind (therefore vata) more and takes the emphasis away from the intellect.

---

[1] *Astanga Hrdayam*, vols; I - III, trans. Murthy, Prof. K.R. Srikantha, Varanasi, India; Krishnadas Academy, 3rd ed. 1996 Vol. I pg. 24

11 Snehana and Other Methods

"Therefore one should always inquire into the nature of the world, the individual Self and the supreme Self. When the ideas of the individual Self and the world are negated, the pure, supreme Self alone remains."
—Pancadasi, VI-12

Snehana is very different than Abhyanga in that technique is of little importance. It primarily uses oil and herbs as a therapeutic medium with the activating kind of stroke. The primary application of Snehana is in the Pancha Karma method of treatment. We can use Snehana outside of Pancha Karma to treat vata disorders and to drive the humors back to their homes. The pacifying of the vata dosha and the diseases that it causes is the main use of Snehana outside of Pancha Karma. The other main application of Snehana is very deep connective tissue work which requires some preparation of the client before treatment. There other uses but they are from a purely medical point of view and need to be prescribed by an Ayurvedic doctor.

The preparations to give Snehana are more complicated in that they require a method to contain, or to contain and recycle, the oil used. It is typical to use between 2 to 4 quarts of oil in a session. Usually the oil is applied by one person and two massage therapists rub the oil into the patient vigorously, one on each side. Sometimes four therapists are used, two for the upper body and two for the legs. This is how it is done in many parts of India.

It is possible to use Snehana in the West, but most people will find it awkward and very messy. I have adapted it somewhat in the exercise outlined below.

Practice Exercises for Snehana

1. Prepare the floor to work on by spreading a large sheet of plastic over the work area. A good size is about 10' x 15'. This way you can roll up the edges a bit to keep extra oil from flowing off the plastic (tuck the edges under so that it makes a curb of sorts). Over this lay a cotton sheet that you don't mind losing. No pillows or cushions are used. The floor will be hard.

2. Choose a medicated oil that suites your client, have at least two quarts available.

3. If deeper connective tissue is going to be the main focus then your client should be prepared one week in advance internally. This is accomplished by drinking a 1/2 cup of oil (as per constitution and perhaps with herbs like ginger) twice per day, morning and evening. This must be done according to the constitution and the digestive ability (agni) of the person. An Ayurvedic doctor should be consulted for this method as there are many restrictions associated to internal oleation therapy. However, this lubricates the intestinal system and causes a purge of sorts. The client should be warned that they may have diarrhea. The oil will penetrate all seven tissue levels in the seven days, providing lubrication from the inside. If this is not done then deep connective tissue work should not be attempted from the point of view of Ayurveda. This is like using a dirty rag to clean the table (as is often the case in India!). The vessel, or body, must be prepared before one can expect a good result. This is described in ancient texts as a dried stick of wood being bent until it breaks. Or taking the same stick and soaking it in oil for a week and then bending it; it will not break. The founders of Ayurveda are not stupid, they know that by oiling the inside first miracles are possible in bodywork. Ayurveda always states that one must purify the body before strengthening the patient, this also applies to deep tissue work. Hence, during the week of preparation the person should also follow a sattvic, or light eliminating diet. Improper preparation sets the stage for therapeutic failure.

4. The client should lay flat on the sheet facing the ceiling. In some schools the back is not done at all. I feel that it should

always be done. But start on the front of the body.

5. Begin with the head. Pour oil over the forehead with your right hand, lay the edge of your left hand on their eyebrows (just above) to prevent the oil from entering into the patients eyes. Their head should be slightly tilted backwards to help the oil avoid the eyes and to allow the oil to enter their hair. Pour one cup of warm oil very slowly in this manner over the center of the forehead, or the Sthapani marma (N° 4). Let the oil run into the hair.

6. Pour more oil into the hair until it is oily and massage the head with vigorous circular movements. Cover the whole head in this manner. Use more oil if needed.

7. Begin now with the activating kind of stroke on the shoulders, moving down the arm first, then the whole side of the body as in the previous method. The difference here is that you must pour oil on the body constantly. One cup of oil per quarter of the body is about right. You will need more for the hands and feet. The front of the body should be rubbed well. Start from the top and go all the way through to the foot, then do the other side.

8. Now roll the patient over and do the back in the same manner. Be sure that you are putting enough oil on that it pools or runs off. Your strokes must be fast enough to catch the oil and keep it mostly on the body (although in India it is allowed to run off freely).

9. When both sides are done roll the patient back over and start deep tissue work or just repeat step 7.

10. Now do deep tissue work or repeat step 8.

11. As the floor is hard, the person will be somewhat uncomfortable. This will effect vata types the most and so they should not be kept as long in one position as the others, kapha has the most resistance and should be kept uncomfortable longer and the work should go deeper. Vata types should have an equal amount of time on the front and back of the body as on their hands and feet. Pitta more on the body, kapha needs very little on the hands and feet. Finish with the hands and feet according to constitution.

12. In some cases kapha types need to have powder applied to prevent congestion in the body. These cases involve obesity, poor circulation, low blood pressure, water retention, weak kidneys, and general sluggishness. If these apply to your patient rub vigorously a heating herb into their skin to absorb the remaining oil before stopping. Usually these kind of clients should not be given this kind of treatment without the guidance of a doctor.

13. Allow the patient to rest for five minutes on the floor and then have them take a hot shower or bath to wash off excess oil that still remains.

Snehana is not recommended for persons suffering from any kind of congestive disorder (kapha type diseases), nor for people with low agni (digestive power) as it will further suppress the digestion. Snehana should mainly be done with healthy people, very weak or very sick, very young or very old people should not be given this kind of therapy. A light sattvic diet should be maintained by all patients for two weeks after treatment.

Self Healing Massage Techniques

Abhyanga is also the self care kind of massage that each of us should do daily. For this kind of treatment sesame oil is generally used. Abhyanga in this context is used to keep vata in balance and so is usually prescribed to people with vata prakruti. However, I have observed that 80% of my clients suffer from some kind of imbalance of vata. Thus, I feel that most people can benefit from this self care method. Kapha people should refer to Dr. Joshi's book on Pancha Karma[1] for other possible methods to use on self care. Another general reference for all constitutions in this regard is Dr. Frawley's book[2] which also covers diet and herbs.

Oil should be applied warm or hot (not burning). This can be accomplished by putting the bottle of oil in boiling water, or on your heater (if it is winter, for those on Maui use the sun!)

1. Apply oil to your head, massaging the face, ears and neck. Massage the base of your skull without oiling your hair much.

2. Massage your shoulders and lower neck. Rub the oil in with firm strokes.

3. Rub the oil into your arms using straight firm movements. Use circular movements on the joints.

4. Cover your upper body with oil, be careful not to apply more than can be absorbed easily.

5. Do your legs and knees. Massage the bottoms of your feet.

6. Take a hot shower or bath, allowing the oil to penetrate deeper. After the shower or bath wipe off any remaining oil with a towel, avoid using soap as it steals the natural oils from the body.

An alternate method is to take a hot shower and then apply small amounts of sesame oil all over the body. As the pores have been opened by the hot water the oil can penetrate deeper. The oil can then be left on the body and allowed to soak in over time. This method is not as effective as the other, but may be more practical for many people.

Tradition recommends that the sesame oil be cured by heating it to a temperature of 180° F, but not boiling it. It states that this allows for the oil to be absorbed easier. I have not noticed a difference in this regard. In fact, I find that cold pressed, organic sesame oil is absorbed in five minutes if excessive amounts are not applied. This may be due more to the different kinds of oils or preparations than anything. It also varies a lot depending on your constitution. The kind of oils that I find in France may be different than those of the USA or other countries so a person should experiment, if the oil is not penetrating then use the traditional method to 'cure' the oil. Be careful not to overheat or to catch the oil on fire as it is flammable; use only small amounts.

Daily foot massage should be a part of everyone's daily care. Foot massage helps maintain eyesight and hearing, it calms the mind, promotes sleep, it prevent sciatica, and promotes blood circulation in the legs. It is an easy way to calm and maintain the vata dosha.

Practice Exercise for Treating the Five Vayus

This kind of massage also falls under Abhyanga. With it one can work on the natural pranic currents as they flow in the body. In fact, all of the methods described in this book work on the five vayus. Anytime that you touch the lower half of the body from the navel down you are working directly on the apana vayu. When you work on the navel area you are working directly on the samana vayu. When you work on the chest area you are working the prana and vyana vayus. By massaging the throat area you work on the udana vayu. And lastly, by massaging the head you are working directly on the prana vayu, the chief vayu.

In fact any kind of touch or massage primarily relates to the vyana vayu as that is the vayu that controls circulation, relates to the nervous system and the sense of touch. One can say in all honesty that massage in general is directly treating the vyana vayu. Any kind of imbalance usually involves the apana vayu, so all massage can be said to work directly on the apana. Vata relates closest to apana in its imbalanced state.

When working on the pranic currents one must have a certain self-development or self-awareness of your own prana. This is a kind of prerequisite for the practitioner. It is possible to still use these methods without having developed your own prana, but you will be unaware of what is actually happening in your client. This is obvious from the many systems of 'energetic' healing that abound today. While many of them are OK as far as systems go, the practitioners are seldom aware of what they are doing. I am speaking therapeutically here and in the context of Ayurveda and its understanding of the subtle anatomy. From this point of view it is imperative that the therapist train themselves correctly before embarking with a new method. This preparation is your own internal awareness of prana.

One way to learn this is by doing. It is not my intention to put people off or exaggerate the difficulties of working directly on the five vayus. Rather, it is to present the methods according to their tradition and correct utilization. You can easily go through these methods, they are not difficult in their external movements. But this will not be working on the pranas.

The only effective way to treat prana directly is not to think or have any preconceived idea in your mind. Any concept that you are holding effectively restricts or directs the prana that flows from you into your client. The best way to approach these exercises is to first have control over your mind. Or as I proposed before, to be in communion with the pranas and allow them to function through you.

Many 'new age' therapists talk about having the 'energy flow through' into the patient. While this sounds nice, it is seldom the case as this can only happen when your mind is still; i.e., no movement of thought. Otherwise your thoughts are constantly influencing the prana and changing its quality. Not thinking comes about gradually by meditational practices that do not bind one in the trinity of meditator, meditation and the object being meditated on. When this kind of self maturity is present then working on the five vayus gives excellent results and is pleasing for both the practitioner and patient. Having said this I encourage everyone to try these methods and learn from experience. Prana reveals itself to a humble person. When it reveals itself your work becomes easy.

All of these steps are aided and rendered more effective when the therapist consciously projects prana into the patient during the massage. This is not mandatory, only more efficient therapeutically.

1. Begin with yourself. Relax and meditate before your client comes.

2. Do a diagnosis. If vata is at all imbalanced then this kind of treatment is appropriate.

3. Have the client lay down and make them comfortable.

4. Warm sesame oil is the best for this kind of treat-

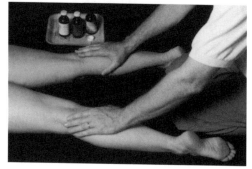

Fig. 40

ment, mixed with ashwagandha and/ or calamus is the best.

5. Begin with the prana that is usually behind all disease - apana vayu. Apana likes to go everywhere other than down, which is its proper place. Start with the feet. Massage them well with warm oil, moving slowly upward on each leg. I prefer to do one leg at a time. When both legs are done do them at the same time (see fig. 40). You are driving the apana back up to the colon, its home. Use enough oil that the patient is well lubricated, push the apana gently up to the colon area with sattvic touch and harmonizing strokes (in this case not circular). When the colon area is reached

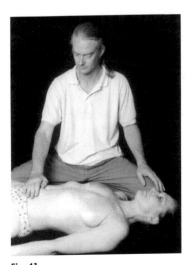

Fig. 41

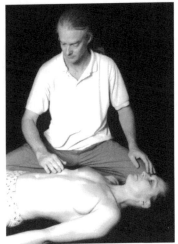

Fig. 42

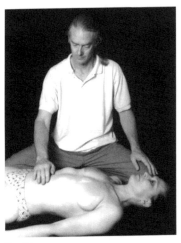

Fig. 43

use more oil and circular, harmonizing massage in a clockwise motion. Stay in the area between the pubic bone and the navel (see fig. 41).

6. Now go to the shoulders and make long, smooth, harmonizing strokes towards the pubic area below the navel. Use enough oil to lubricate the skin well; keep it warm. This will bring apana down to its home area. Repeat this four or five times, or until you feel the apana is down again. When the colon area is reached use more oil and repeat the circular, harmonizing massage in a clockwise motion.

7. Next work on the samana vayu. Samana comes from the periphery to the center. Start from the sides and bring all of your massage strokes to the navel area, the home of samana (see fig. 42). Then start from the shoulders and

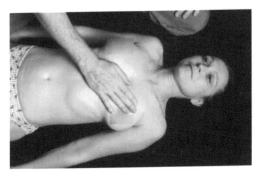

Fig. 44

Secrets of Ayurvedic Massage

bring your strokes to the navel. Then do the legs, starting from the feet and ending at the navel. This brings samana back home to the navel. Now do a clockwise circular massage on the navel (see fig. 43).

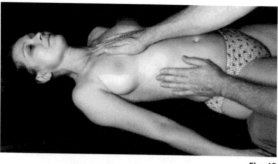

Fig. 45

8. Vyana vayu moves from the center out to the skin and collects in the joints. Start by harmonizing circular massage over the heart area (see fig. 44). When you feel the vyana is calm, let your circles grow until this movement is as big as you can make it on the

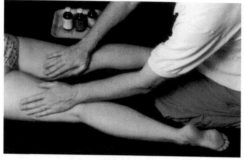

Fig. 46

body (see fig. 45). Then go out to the limbs with small circular movements until all four have been covered (see fig. 46). Pay special attention to the joints. Use enough oil to keep the body well lubricated.

9. Udana moves upward and is our inspiration. When you work on your own prana you are developing your udana. Begin with the 'neck release' technique that was

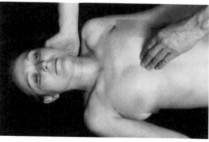

Fig. 47

outlined in Chapter Ten. This works directly to harmonize the udana. When the neck is done place one hand (right) on the sternum and the other (left) on the base of the skull. Wait for five of your own breathing cycles (see fig. 47). Now massage the base of the collar bone with small clockwise movements to harmonize udana (see fig. 48).

10. Prana vayu is best treated by massaging the temples and the marmas associated with them; then the third eye area in the center of the forehead. Use small, harmonizing, clockwise move-

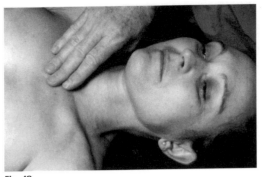
Fig. 48

ments with oil (see fig. 49). Now place one hand on the forehead and one under the head at the base of the skull (see fig. 50). Stay like this for five breathing cycles. Now remove the hand from under the base of the skull and place it on the heart area (see fig. 51).

Stay like this for five breathing cycles or until you feel the prana vayu is in harmony.

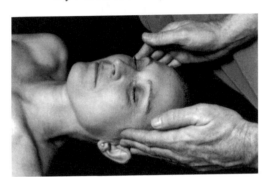
Fig. 49

11. Now lay one hand on the area of apana - between the pubic bone and the navel - and one on the heart. Stay like this until you feel the apana and prana vayus are balanced, or five breathing cycles.

This is a simple method that follows the natural movements of the five vayus. Many other methods are possible, but I favor this as following what the body is already doing - thus, less intrusive. With practice and sensitivity you will be able to feel the subtle currents. Perhaps you may be lucky and the prana will reveal itself to you, in which case your life and work will change completely.

The Practice of No Method

After learning the subtle anatomy, diagnosis, the therapeutic properties of the oils and herbs that you use, and Ayurvedic theory, you may forget them all completely. Once it becomes part of you there will be no need to think of it at all. You can simply forget about it and work completely intuitively. This is perhaps the best method in all forms of bodywork. However, too often the practitioner will want to start here rather than end here.

Ayurveda is a life time study. Ayur is life. Life is not fixed or ever completely knowable. This is why a solid therapeutic system should be your foundation. Ayurveda provides the most comprehensive health care system available in the world. Make it your foundation. When this is done then you can let your hands guide you in your work. This is what my first teacher in massage taught me. Yet, it

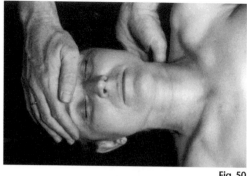

Fig. 50

took years of learning a medical system that could provide the foundation for this intuitive work to really flower. Of course, I *did* start the wrong way myself.

By adding the knowledge and experience that Ayurveda has, your work can improve dramatically. The time and effort to learn Ayurveda will repay itself thousands of times over in your own health

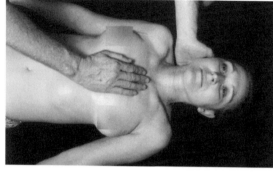

Fig. 51

care and the improved treatment quality to your clients. I advise you in this way because I made these mistakes myself already and having learned the hard way I can warn you of the possible pitfalls.

The best 'method' to use 'no method' is to first have a solid base in Ayurveda. The next is to not think during your sessions. This means no concepts or ideas about your work or your client. This is also called 'being present'. Your presence is by far the most important factor in all forms of bodywork. If this book gives no other message to you than this - be 100% present when you work - then it is a success. This 'presence' is the flowering of Ayurveda and of your own intuitive creativity. The healing arts offer a beautiful outlet for your creativity. This is in fact the tragedy of today's medical system.

This is the very reason why Ayurveda is making a return and why it has survived for so many thousands of years - because it encourages your own creativity to express itself. The exact opposite attitude has been prevalent in modern medicine for the last several centuries. To such an extent that doctors are persecuted by their own colleagues if they are creative and innovative. The vast majority of doctors are not present with their clients, and the clients sense it. They are no better than machines. Occasionally, this attitude has entered massage therapy. Fortunately, this trend is now beginning to change. Ayurveda can provide the comprehensive, logical and flexible system needed to allow a new medical renaissance to appear in the world. Become a part of it for yourself and for your patient's.

Allowing your hands to work and to let your deeper consciousness do the session is the goal of all forms of modern bodywork. The key to this flowering is your own mind and self development. The key in this process it the prana. This is why I have presented so much information on prana. Once you are well versed in the Ayurvedic therapeutic approach you can, through communion, allow the pranas to do the work. This then will give a true quality of healing that one may call love.

[1] Joshi, Dr. Sunil V., *Ayurveda and Panchakarma*, Twin Lakes, WI; Lotus Press, 1996
[2] Frawley, Dr. David, *Ayurvedic Healing: A Comprehensive Guide*, Salt Lake City, UT: Passage Press, 1989

Appendix 1 **Marma Points**

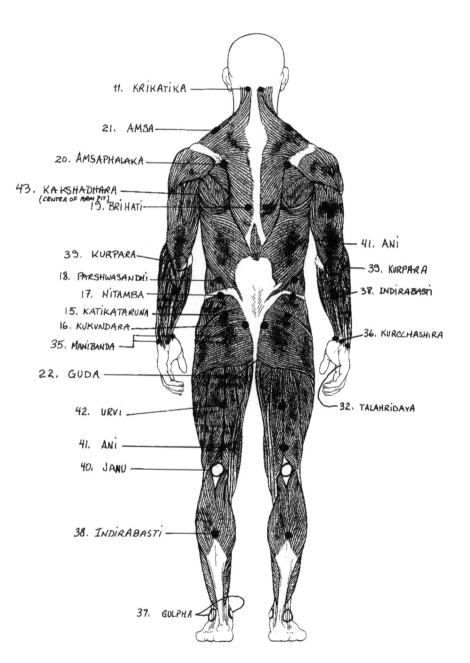

11. KRIKATIKA

21. AMSA

20. AMSAPHALAKA

43. KAKSHADHARA
(CENTER OF ARM PIT)

19. BRIHATI

39. KURPARA

18. PARSHWASANDHI

17. NITAMBA

15. KATIKATARUNA

16. KUKUNDARA

35. MANIBANDA

22. GUDA

42. URVI

41. ANI

40. JANU

38. INDIRABASTI

37. GULPHA

41. ANI

39. KURPARA

38. INDIRABASTI

36. KURCCHASHIRA

32. TALAHRIDAYA

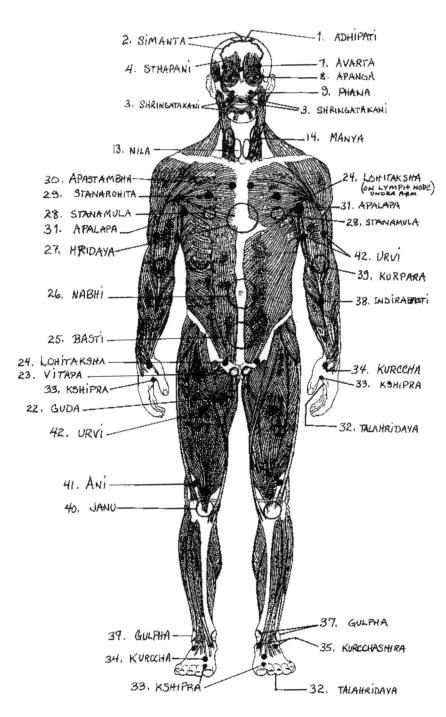

2. SIMANTA
1. ADHIPATI
4. STHAPANI
7. AVARTA
8. APANGA
9. PHANA
3. SHRINGATAKANI
3. SHRINGATAKANI
14. MANYA
13. NILA
30. APASTAMBHA
29. STANAROHITA
24. LOHITAKSHA (ON LYMPH NODE UNDER ARM)
31. APALAPA
28. STANAMULA
28. STANAMULA
31. APALAPA
42. URVI
27. HRIDAYA
39. KURPARA
26. NABHI
38. INDIRABASTI
25. BASTI
24. LOHITAKSHA
23. VITAPA
34. KURCCHA
33. KSHIPRA
33. KSHIPRA
22. GUDA
42. URVI
32. TALAHRIDAYA
41. ANI
40. JANU
37. GULPHA
39. GULPHA
35. KURCCHASHIRA
34. KURCCHA
33. KSHIPRA
32. TALAHRIDAYA

Appendix 2

Bibliograhy

Astanga Hrdayam, vols; I - III, trans. Murthy, Prof. K.R. Srikantha, Varanasi, India; Krishnadas Academy, 3rd ed. 1996

Atreya, *Practical Ayurveda: Secrets of Physical, Sexual & Spiritual Health*, York Beach, Me; Samuel Weiser, Inc. 1998

_____, *Prana: The Secret of Yogic Healing*, York Beach, Me; Samuel Weiser, Inc. 1996

Clifford, Terry, *Tibetan Buddhist Medicine and Psychiatry*, York Beach, ME: Samuel Weiser Inc., 1984

Dash, Dr. Bhagwan & Sharma, Dr. R.K., *Caraka Samhita*, Varanasi, India: Chowkamba Series Office, 1992, 3 vols.

Dash, Dr. Bhagwan, *Massage Therapy in Ayurveda*, New Delhi, India: Concept Publishing Co., 1992

_____, *Five Specialised Therapies of Ayurveda*, New Delhi, India: Concept Publishing Co., 1992

_____, *Ayurvedic Cures For Common Diseases*, Delhi, India: Hind Pocket Books, 1993 4th ed.

_____, *Madanapala's Nighantu - Materia Medica*, New Delhi, India: B. Jain Publishers, 1991

_____, *Ayurveda Saukhyam of Todarananda - Materia Medica*, New Delhi, India: Concept Publishing Co., 1980

Devaraj, Dr. T.L., *Speaking of: Ayurvedic Remedies for Common Diseases*, New Delhi, India: Sterling Publishers, 1985

Eight Upanishads, vols. I & II, trans. Swami Gambhirananda, Calcuta, India: Advaita Ashrama, 1992

Frawley, Dr. David, *Ayurvedic Healing: A Comprehensive Guide*, Salt Lake City, UT: Passage Press, 1989

_____, *Tantric Yoga and the Wisdom Goddesses*, Salt Lake City, UT: Passage Press, 1994

_____, *Ayurveda and the Mind; The Healing of Consciousness*, Twin Lakes, WI: Lotus Press, 1997

_____, *Astrology of the Seers*, Salt Lake City, UT: Passage Press, 1990

_____, *Gods, Sages and Kings; Vedic Secrets of Ancient Civilization*, Salt Lake City, UT: Passage Press, 1991

_____, & Lad, Dr. Vasant, *The Yoga of Herbs*, Twin Lakes, WI: Lotus Press, 1986

Heyn, Birgit, *Ayurvedic Medicine: The Gentle Strength of Indian Healing*, New Delhi, India: Indus - HarperCollins India, 1992

Johari, Harish, *Ayurvedic Massage*, Rochester, VT; Healing Arts Press, 1996

Joshi, Dr. Sunil V., *Ayurveda and Panchakarma*, Twin Lakes, WI; Lotus Press, 1996

Lad, Dr. Vasant, *Ayurveda: The Science of Self-Healing*, Twin Lakes, WI: Lotus Press, 1984

_____, *Secrets of the Pulse*, Albuquerque, NM: The Ayurvedic Institute, 1996

_____, & Frawley, Dr. David, *The Yoga of Herbs*, Twin Lakes, WI: Lotus Press, 1986

_____, & Lad, Usha, *Ayurvedic Cooking for Self-Healing*, Twin Lakes, WI: Lotus Press, 1994

Miller, Dr. Light & Dr. Bryan, *Ayurveda & Aromatherapy*, Twin Lakes, WI: Lotus Press, 1995

Morningstar, Amadea, *The Ayurvedic Cookbook*, Twin Lakes, WI: Lotus Press, 1990

_____, *Ayurvedic Cooking for Westerners*, Twin Lakes, WI: Lotus Press, 1994

Nisargadatta, Maharaj, *I Am That*, Bombay, India: Chetana Ltd., 1991

_____, *Prior To Consciousness* Durham, NC: Acorn Press, 1985

_____, *Seeds Of Consciousness*, Durham, NC: Acorn Press, 1990

_____, *Consciousness And The Absolute*, Durham, NC: Acorn Press, 1994

Pancadasi, Vidyaranya Swami, Madras, India, Ramakrishna Math, 1987

Poonja, Sri H.W.L., *The Truth Is*, San Anselmo, CA: Vidya Sagar Publications, 1998

_____, *Wake Up And Roar*, Vols. I & II, Kula, Maui, Hawaii: Pacific Center Pub, 1992

_____, *Papaji*, Ed. David Godman, Boulder, CO: Avadhuta Foundation, 1993

Ranade, Dr. Subhash, *Natural Healing Through Ayurveda*, Salt Lake City, UT: Passage Press, 1993

Ramana Maharishi, *Be As You Are*, Ed. David Godman, New Delhi, India: Penguin Books India, 1992

_____, *Talks With Sri Ramana Maharishi*, Trans. Swami Ramanananda, Tiruvannamalai, India: Sri Ramanasramam, 1984

Ramanananda, Swami, Trans., *Advaita Bodha Deepika*, Tiruvannamalai, India: Sri Ramanasramam, 1990

_____, Trans., *Tripura Rahasya*, Tiruvannamalai, India: Sri Ramanasramam, 1989

Ros, Dr. Frank, *The Lost Secrets of Ayurvedic Acupuncture*, Twin Lakes, WI: Lotus Press, 1994

Sachs, Melanie, *Ayurvedic Beauty Care*, Lotus Press, WI: Twin Lakes, 1994

Sharma, Dr. Priya Vrat, *Sodasangahrdayam - Essentials of Ayurveda*, Delhi, India: Motilal Banarsidass Publishers, 1993

Svoboda, Dr. Robert, *Prakruti: Your Ayurvedic Constitution*, Albuquerque, NM: Geocom Ltd., 1989

_____, *Ayurveda: Life, Health and Longevity*, New Delhi, India: Penguin Books India, 1993

_____, *Aghora: At the Left Hand of God*, Albuquerque, NM: Brotherhood of Life Publishing, 1986

_____, *Aghora II: Kundalini, Albuquerque*, NM: Brotherhood of Life Publishing, 1993

_____, *Aghora III: The Law of Karma*, Albuquerque, NM: Brotherhood of Life Publishing, 1997

Tierra, Michael, *Planetary Herbology*, Twin Lakes, WI: Lotus Press, 1988

_____, *The Way of Herbs*, New York, NY: Pocket Books, 1980

Tiwari, Maya, *Ayurveda: Secrets of Healing*, Twin Lakes, WI; Lotus Press, 1995

Vanhowten, Donald, *Ayurveda & Life Impressions Bodywork*, Twin Lakes, WI; Lotus Press, 1997

Yoga Vasistha, "The Supreme Yoga" Vols. I & II, Swami Venkatesananda trans., Shivanandanagar, Uttar Pradesh, India: Divine Life Society, 1991

Appendix 3

Glossary

Abhyanga: therapeutic or daily massage

Agni: first of three cosmic principals; god of fire; digestive fire.

Allopathy: western medicine, modern medicine.

Apana prana: one of the five pranas; the prana that controls all evacuation, called the downward breath; resides in the lower abdomen.

Aphrodisiac: any substance that promotes health to the reproductive organs.

Ashram: place devoted to spiritual development (though rarely is!).

Astanga Hrdayam: one of the three ancient Ayurvedic texts of medicine.

Atma: consciousness or God in an individualized sense.

Ayurveda: The oldest medical system in the world. A holistic approach developed by the same sages who formed the systems of yoga. The part of the Vedas dealing with the health of the body; the science of life.

Brimhana: strengthening or fortifying therapies in Ayurveda.

Brahma: consciousness in an absolute sense; one of the three aspects of consiousness, the creator or creative aspect; the founder of Ayurveda in the form of a god.

Brahman: is a term used to describe that which is not possible to describe, it is often just called - being, conscious, bliss, or sat, chit, anand; the Self

Brahmin: the learned class of people in Vedic society; priests.

Bramhacharya: abidance in Brahma or the unmanifest reality.

Caraka Samhita: the oldest surviving text of Ayurveda; one of the three ancient Ayurvedic texts of medicine.

Chi: Chinese word for Prana.

Chit: consciousness

Consciousness: as used in this book, the Substratum or Source of all manifestation.

Constitution: an individuals unique mix of the three humors.

Dhatu: tissue; there are seven different tissue levels in Ayurveda - plasma, blood, muscle, fat, bone, bone marrow and nerve tissue, and reproductive fluids.

Dosha: Sanskrit for humor; lit: that which will imbalance or 'fault'.

Energetic Impressions: in Sanskrit there are two kinds: Vasanas & Samskaras, these are latent, unconscious or stored impressions and current mental impressions; these impressions are stored in the subtle body; Yoga says that these impressions are what cause us to incarnate in another life, unless they are allowed to surface to consciousness; these impressions along with prana create what we call mind.

Inquiry: method to find out where thoughts, prana arise from; question: "Who am I?"; see books of Ramana Maharishi and H.W.L. Poonjaji.

Five elements: the five states of material existence: mass, liquidity, transformation, movement, and the field in which they function; also called: earth, water, fire, air, & ether.

Five states of matter: commonly called the Five Elements.

Ghee: butter that has gone through a process of cooking to render it free from deterioration; used for cooking and as a vehicle for herbal medicines.

Guna: quality, attribute of intelligence; there are three gunas: sattva, rajas, and tamas; therapeutically it is the quality of a herb or substance, i.e., oily, slimy, dry, etc.

Guru: Lit. dispeller of ignorance; one who knows the substratum or source of creation; teacher; heavy.

Humor: a unique concept to describe the functions of the body; the forces which balance the five elements together in the body; there are three humors: vata (wind), pitta (fire), and kapha (water). There is a fourth humor called the 'sense of humor' which is often lacking in people - it is worthwhile to develop.

Kapha: one of the three humors; controls water and earth elements.

Karma: action; the cosmic law of for every action there is a reaction; there is no such thing as "bad or good" karma; therapeutically it is the general action of a herb or substance in the body.

Ki: Japanese word for prana.

Kundalini: the primordial prana that rests dormant in the body unless activated by special practices; NOTE: these practices are dangerous unless one is supervised by a qualified teacher.

Langhana: reducing therapies in Ayurveda

Latent impression: see Energetic impressions.

Life Force: another name of prana, especially those five in the body.

Mantra: the science of sound; by using the correct sound each prana can be harmonized - and so the mind.

Marma: a sensitive point of the body that stimulates the pranic flow; the acupressure and acupuncture points of Ayurveda.

Maya: the illusion that everything exists as separate from God.

Meridians: the channels of prana in the body; called nadis in yoga.

Mind: thoughts moving through consciousness, giving the illusion of continuity; the combination of prana and vasanas.

Nadi: see meridian.

No-Mind: non movement of thought; complete awareness; not to be confused with the Absolute, the individual may still exist at this point, it may take many times of being emerged in no-mind before the individual dissolves into pure consciousness.

Ojas: the essence of food; the basis of the immune system; we are born with eight drops of ojas in the heart center, if this is reduced, death results; there is a secondary ojas which is the result of all the tissue elements, it can vary in quantity, however, when it is reduced sickness results (ref.: Caraka Samhita Vol. I Pg. 594).

Pancha Karma: the Five Actions; five reducing therapies in Ayurveda.

Parabdha: the karma or action that is residual; the karma's associated with the body/mind manifestation, in other words as long as you have a body the Parabdha karma continues.

Pitta: one of the three humors; controls fire and water elements.

Prakriti: the dynamic energy of consciousness; natal constitution; nature.

Prana: pra = before, ana = breath; the vital force; vayu; Qi, Ki, Chi; it arises from substratum of pure consciousness with intelligence (agni) and love (soma) together they create the individualized consciousness. There are five major pranas in the human body, prana, apana, samana, udana and vyana, they arise from the cosmic prana and the rajas guna; chief of the five pranas in the body, called the outward going breath, it resides in the head and the heart.

Pranayama: A method of breath control used to regulate the mind and the prana, thereby the physical and mental health. Should only be practiced with a qualified teacher.

Pranic healing: a therapeutic method that harmonizes the pranas directly.

Purusha: the unmanifest aspect of consciousness; the void.

Qi: another name of prana.

Rajas: one of the three gunas; action, movement, bright, energy, aggression, aggravated mind, achievement, and strong emotions.

Rama: the disciple of Vasistha and the student that receives the teaching in the Yoga Vasistha; avatar; one of the manifestations of Vishnu, the force of preservation in the universe; the hero of the epic poem Ramayana; pure consciousness embodied.

Samana prana: one of the five pranas in the body; called the equalizing prana it resides in the navel region.

Samsara: the concept that we are separate from God; suffering; illusion.

Samskaras: Innate energetic impressions, see energetic impressions.

Sattva: one of the three gunas; purity, peace, calm, beauty, happiness, quiet obedient mind, and stable emotions.

Sattvic diet: a diet that promotes Sattva; very mild nourishing foods like milk, basmati rice, mung beans, and fruits.

Self: another name for pure consciousness; also called Brahman or the substratum of all duality- ie, creation; our true nature, hence the term -"self".

Shakti: cosmic prana.

Shiva: pure consciousness; one of the three aspects of consciousness as god, the destroyer.

Sidhi: psychic powers.

Snehana: massage using oils as part of oleation therapy; generally used as preparation for Pancha Karma.

Soma: nectar; the most subtle essence of ojas and kapha; the God Soma signifies love, unity.

Srotas: channels in the Ayurvedic system that carry substances like blood, air, and thought.

Substratum: equal to: The Absolute, pure Consciousness, Love, Brahman, Atman, Self, or Source.

Sushruta Samhita: one of the three ancient Ayurvedic texts of medicine.

Tamas: one of the three gunas; inertia, dull, depressed, void, stupid, lazy, despair, and self destructive emotions.

Tantra: A path that totally accepts all aspects of the physical world, believing that all things lead to the divine; worship of the divine mother; often confused as a sexual practice.

Taste: the beginning of the therapeutic actions of any substance on the body.

Tejas: the subtle form of pitta; the power of discrimination in the mind.

Trikutu: a famous Ayurvedic formula that stimulates digestion and agni; very good for kapha.

Triphala: a famous Ayurvedic formula for rejuvenating the body, promoting digestion, and harmonizing all the digestive organs.

Udana prana: one of the five pranas in the body; called the upward moving breath, it is seated in the throat; kundalini yoga cultivates this prana as do all psychic powers.

Vakruti: the constitution of the moment; that which covers prakruti.

Vasanas: Latent energetic impression, see energetic impressions.

Vasishta: the most prominent sage in the Vedas; one of the seven immortal seers; the source of the Yoga Vasishta.

Vata: one of the three humors; controls wind (air) and ether elements.

Vayu: the God of the Wind; another name for Vata; another name for prana.

Vedas: Literally it means knowledge, but used here to mean the Book of Knowledge, the oldest book in the world; there are four Vedas.

Vipaka: the long term effect of an herb or substance.

Virya: the potency (hot or cold) of an herb or substance.

Vishnu: consciousness as pure love; the aspect of consciousness that protects and preserves the world; as a god he has seven main manifestations of which Rama and Krishna are the two most famous.

Vyana prana: one of the five pranas in the body; called the equalizing breath it unifies all the other pranas and the body, it is diffused throughout the body.

Yantra: a sound or syllable transformed into a geometric form, usually inscribed in a metal plate or in stone.

Yoga: Union. That which leads one back to the original Source; generally understood to mean a path or a practice leading to the Divine; not limited to Hatha yoga or asanas.

Appendix 4

Herb Glossary

ALPHABETICAL BY LATIN NAMES

Latin	Indian	English
Acora calamus	Vacha	Calamus
Aegle marmelos	Bilva	none
Asafoetida	Hing	Asafoetida
Asparagus adscendens	Safed Mushali	White Asparagus
Asparagus racemosus	Shatavri	Asparagus
Asphaltum	Shilajit	Mineral Pitch
Azadiracta indica	Neem	Neem
Bambusa arundinacia	Vamsha Rochana	Bamboo Manna
Berberis arista	Daru Haldi	Wood Turmeric
Boerhaavia diffusa	Punarnava	Hog weed
Brassica alba	Svetasarisha	Mustard (White)
Caryophyllus aromaticus	Lavanga	Clove
Cinnamomum zeylanicum	Dalchini	Cinnamon
Cinnamomum iners	Tejpatra	Tamala
Cocus nucifera	Tranaraj	Coconut
Convolvolos pluricaulis	Shankpushpi	Shankpushpi
Commiphora mukul	Guggulu	Guggulu
Coriandrum sativum	Dhanyaka	Coriander
Crocus sativus	Kesar	Saffron
Cumimum cyminum	Safed Jerra	White Cumin
Curcuma longa	Haldi	Turmeric
Cyperus rotundus	Musta	Nut Grass
Eclipta alba	Bhringraj	Eclipta
Ellataria cardamomum	Elacihi	Cardamom
Emblica officinalis	Amalaki	Indian Gooseberry
Embelia ribes	Vidanga	Embelia
Foeniculum vulgare	Bari Saunf	Fennel
Glycyrrhiza glabra	Mulethi	Licorice
Helianthus annuus	Arkakantha	Sunflower

Hemidesmus indicus	Anantmool	Indian Sarsaparilla
Hydrocotyle asiatica	Brahmi	Gotu Kola
Mucuna pruriens	Kaunch	Cowhage
Myristica fragrans	Jaiphal	Nutmeg
Nardostachys jatamansi	Jatamansi	Spikenard
Nelumbo nucifera	Kamal Bees	Lotus Seeds
Nigella sativa	Kali Jerra	Black Cumin
Ocimum sanctum	Tulsi	Holy Basil
Olea europaea	none	Olive
Picrorrhiza kurroa	Kutki	Picrorrhiza
Piper longum	Pippli	Long Pepper
Piper nigrum	Kalimirch	Black Pepper
Plumbago zeylanica	Chitrak	Ceylon Leadwort
Polygonatum officinale	Meda	Solomon Seal
Pterocarpus santalinus	Rakta Chandana	Red Sandalwood
Prunus amygdalus	Badam	Almond
Ricinus communis	Eranda	Castor bean or oil
Rubia cordifolia	Manjishta	Indian Madder
Santalum alba	Chandana	Sandalwood
Sesamun indicum	Tila	Sesame
Sida cordifolia	Bala	Country Mallow
Solanum indicum	Brihati	none
Swertia chirata	Chiraita	Indian Gentian
Terminalia belerica	Bibhitaki	Beleric myrobalan
Terminalia chebula	Haritaki	Chebulic myrobalan
Tinispora cordifolia	Guduchi	Amrita
Tribulis terrestris	Gokshura	Caltrops
Valeriana wallichi	Thagara	Indian Valerian
Withania somnifera	Ashwagandha	Winter Cherry
Zingiber officinale	Sunthi	Ginger
Zea mays	Yavanala	Corn

ALPHABETICAL BY INDIAN NAMES

Emblica officinalis	Amalaki	Indian Gooseberry
Hemidesmus indicus	Anantmool	Indian Sarsaparilla
Helianthus annuus	Arkakantha	Sunflower
Withania somnifera	Ashwagandha	Winter Cherry
Prunus amygdalus	Badam	Almond
Foeniculum vulgare	Bari Saunf	Fennel
Sida cordifolia	Bala	Country Mallow
Eclipta alba	Bhringraj	Eclipta

Secrets of Ayurvedic Massage

Terminalia belerica	Bibhitaki	Beleric myrobalan
Aegle marmelos	Bilva	none
Hydrocotyle asiatica	Brahmi	Gotu Kola
Solanum indicum	Brihati	none
Plumbago zeylanica	Chitrak	Ceylon Leadwort
Santalum alba	Chandana	Sandalwood
Swertia chirata	Chiraita	Indian Gentian
Berberis arista	Daru Haldi	Wood Turmeric
Cinnamomum zeylanicum	Dalchini	Cinnamon
Coriandrum sativum	Dhanyaka	Coriander
Ellataria cardamomum	Elacihi	Cardamom
Ricinus communis	Eranda	Castor bean or oil
Tribulis terrestris	Gokshura	Caltrops
Commiphora mukul	Guggulu	Guggulu
Tinispora cordifolia	Guduchi	Amrita
Curcuma longa	Haldi	Turmeric
Terminalia chebula	Haritaki	Chebulic myrobalan
Asafoetida	Hing	Asafoetida
Myristica fragrans	Jaiphal	Nutmeg
Nardostachys jatamansi	Jatamansi	Spikenard
Nelumbo nucifera	Kamal Bees	Lotus Seeds
Nigella sativa	Kali Jerra	Black Cumin
Piper nigrum	Kalimirch	Black Pepper
Mucuna pruriens	Kaunch	Cowhage
Crocus sativus	Kesar	Saffron
Picrorrhiza kurroa	Kutki	Picrorrhiza
Caryophyllus aromaticus	Lavanga	Clove
Rubia cordifolia	Manjishta	Indian Madder
Polygonatum officinale	Meda	Solomon Seal
Cyperus rotundus	Musta	Nut Grass
Glycyrrhiza glabra	Mulethi	Licorice
Azadiracta indica	Neem	Neem
Piper longum	Pippli	Long Pepper
Boerhaavia diffusa	Punarnava	Hog weed
Pterocarpus santalinus	Rakta Chandana	Red Sandalwood
Asparagus adescendens	Safed Mushali	White Asparagus
Cumimum cyminum	Safed Jerra	White Cumin
Asparagus racemosus	Shatavri	Asparagus
Asphaltum	Shilajit	Mineral Pitch
Convolvolos pluricaulis	Shankpushpi	Shankpushpi
Zingiber officinale	Sunthi	Ginger

Brassica alba	Svetasarisha	Mustard (White)
Cinnamomum iners	Tejpatra	Tamala
Valeriana wallichi	Thagara	Indian Valerian
Sesamun indicum	Tila	Sesame
Cocus nucifera	Tranaraj	Coconut
Ocimum sanctum	Tulsi	Holy Basil
Acora calamus	Vacha	Calamus
Bambusa arundinacia	Vamsha Rochana	Bamboo Manna
Embelia ribes	Vidanga	Embelia
Zea mays	Yavanala	Corn

ALPHABETICAL BY ENGLISH NAMES

Prunus amygdalus	Badam	Almond
Tinispora cordifolia	Guduchi	Amrita
Asafoetida	Hing	Asafoetida
Asparagus racemosus	Shatavri	Asparagus
Bambusa arundinacia	Vamsha Rochana	Bamboo Manna
Terminalia belerica	Bibhitaki	Beleric myrobalan
Nigella sativa	Kali Jerra	Black Cumin
Piper nigrum	Kalimirch	Black Pepper
Acora calamus	Vacha	Calamus
Tribulis terrestris	Gokshura	Caltrops
Ellataria cardamomum	Elacihi	Cardamom
Ricinus communis	Eranda	Castor bean or oil
Plumbago zeylanica	Chitrak	Ceylon Leadwort
Terminalia chebula	Haritaki	Chebulic myrobalan
Cinnamomum zeylanicum	Dalchini	Cinnamon
Caryophyllus aromaticus	Lavanga	Clove
Cocus nucifera	Tranaraj	Coconut
Zea mays	Yavanala	Corn
Coriandrum sativum	Dhanyaka	Coriander
Sida cordifolia	Bala	Country Mallow
Mucuna pruriens	Kaunch	Cowhage
Eclipta alba	Bhringraj	Eclipta
Embelia ribes	Vidanga	Embelia
Foeniculum vulgare	Bari Saunf	Fennel
Zingiber officinale	Sunthi	Ginger
Hydrocotyle asiatica	Brahmi	Gotu Kola
Commiphora mukul	Guggulu	Guggulu
Boerhaavia diffusa	Punarnava	Hog weed

Ocimum sanctum	Tulsi	Holy Basil
Swertia chirata	Chiraita	Indian Gentian
Emblica officinalis	Amalaki	Indian Gooseberry
Rubia cordifolia	Manjishta	Indian Madder
Hemidesmus indicus	Anantmool	Indian Sarsaparilla
Valeriana wallichi	Thagara	Indian Valerian
Glycyrrhiza glabra	Mulethi	Licorice
Nelumbo nucifera	Kamal Bees	Lotus Seeds
Piper longum	Pippli	Long Pepper
Asphaltum	Shilajit	Mineral Pitch
Brassica alba	Svetasarisha	Mustard (White)
Azadiracta indica	Neem	Neem
Cyperus rotundus	Musta	Nut Grass
Myristica fragrans	Jaiphal	Nutmeg
Picrorrhiza kurroa	Kutki	Picrorrhiza
Olea europæa	none	Olive
Pterocarpus santalinus	Rakta Chandana	Red Sandalwood
Crocus sativus	Kesar	Saffron
Santalum alba	Chandana	Sandalwood
Sesamun indicum	Tila	Sesame
Convolvolos pluricaulis	Shankpushpi	Shankpushpi
Polygonatum officinale	Meda	Solomon Seal
Nardostachys jatamansi	Jatamansi	Spikenard
Helianthus annuus	Arkakantha	Sunflower
Cinnamomum iners	Tejpatra	Tamala
Curcuma longa	Haldi	Turmeric
Asparagus adescendens	Safed Mushali	White Asparagus
Cumimum cyminum	Safed Jerra	White Cumin
Withania somnifera	Ashwagandha	Winter Cherry
Berberis arista	Daru Haldi	Wood Turmeric

Appendix 5

Resources

Aromatherapy Video & Home Study Program

Michael Scholes (founder of Aroma Vera)
3384 South Robertson Pl.
Los Angeles, CA 90034
Ph: 800-677-2368

Jeanne Rose Aromatherapy & Herbal Healing Intensives
Attn: Jeanne Rose
219 Carl Street
San Francisco, CA 94117

London School of Aromatherapy
P. O. Box 780
London NW5 1DY
England

Pacific Institute of Aromatherapy
Attn: Kurt Schnaubelt
P. O. Box 8723
San Rafael, CA 94903
Ph: 515-479-9121

Quintessence Aromatherapy
Attn: Ann Berwick
P. O. Box 4996
Boulder, CO 80306
Ph: 303-258-3791

Ayurveda Centers and Programs

Australian Institute of Ayurvedic Medicine
19 Bowey Avenue
Enfield S.A. 5085

Australia
Ph: 08-349-7303

Australian School of Ayurveda
Dr. Krishna Kumar, MD, FIIM
27 Blight Street
Ridleyton, South Australia 5008
Ph. 08-346-0631

Ayur-Veda AB
Box 78, 285 22 Markaryd
Esplanaden 2
Sweden
0433-104 90 (Phone)
0433-104 92 (Fax)
E-Mail: info@ayur-veda.se

Ayurveda for Radiant
Health & Beauty
16 Espira Court
Santa Fe, NM 87505
Ph: 505-466-7662

Ayurvedic Healing Arts Center
16508 Pine Knoll Road
Grass Valley, CA 95945
Ph: 916-274-9000

Ayurvedic Healings
Dr's Light & Bryan Miller
P. O. Box 35214
Sarasota, FL 34242
Ph: 941-346-3581

Ayurvedic Holistic Center
82A Bayville Ave.
Bayville, NY 11709

The Ayurvedic Institute and Wellness Center

11311 Menaul, NE
Albuquerque, NM 87112
Ph: 505-291-9698
Fax: 505-294-7572

Ayurvedic Living Workshops
P.O. Box 188
Exeter, Devon EX4 5AB
England

California College of Ayurveda
1117A East Main Street
Grass Valley, CA 95945
Ph: 530-274-9100
Web: ayurvedacollege.com
E-Mail: info@ayurvedacollege.com
Clinical training in Ayurveda.

Center for Mind, Body Medicine
P. O. Box 1048
La Jolla, CA 92038
Ph: 619-794-2425

The Chopra Center for Well Being
7590 Fay Avenue
Suite 403
LaJolla, CA 92037
Ph: 619-551-7788
Fax: 619-551-7811

John Douillard — Life Spa,
Rejuvenation through Ayur-Veda
3065 Center Green Dr.
Boulder, CO 80301
Ph: 303-442-1164
Fax: 303-442-1240

East West College of Herbalism
Ayurvedic Program
Represents courses of Dr. David
Frawley and Dr. Michael Tierra
in UK
Hartswood, Marsh Green,
Hartsfield
E. Sussex TN7 4ET
United Kingdom
Ph: 01342-822312
Fax: 01342-826346
E-Mail: ewcolherb@aol.com

EverGreen Herb Garden and
Learning Center, Candis

Cantin Packard
P. O. Box 1445,
Placerville CA 95667
Ph. and Fax: 530-626-9288
E-Mail: evrgreen@innercite.com

Himalayan Institute
RR1, Box 400
Honesdale, PA 18431
Ph: 800-822-4547
E-Mail: earthess@aol.com
Web: ayurvedichealing.com

Inside Ayurveda — Bi-monthly,
independent publication for
ayurvedic professionals.
A. Niika Quistgard
P. O. Box 3021
Quincy CA 95971-3021
Ph: 530-283-3717
E-Mail: oflife@inreach.com

Institute for Wholistic Education
33719 116th Street
Box AM
Twin Lakes, WI 53181
Ph: 262-877-9396

Rocky Mountain Ayurveda
Health Retreat
P.O. Box 5192
Pagosa Springs, CO 81147
Ph: 800-247-9654 or 970-264-9224
E-Mail:
valentines@ayurveda-retreat.com
Web: www.ayurveda-retreat.com/
rockymountain

Beginner and Advanced Correspondence Courses in Ayurveda

Integrated Health Systems
3855 Via Nova Marie, #302D
Carmel, CA 93923
Ph: 408-476-5130

International Academy of Ayurved
NandNandan, Atreya Rugnalaya
M.Y. Lele Chowk
Erandawana, Pune: 411 004, India

Ph/Fax: 91-212-378532/524427
E-Mail: avilele@hotmail.com

International Ayurvedic Institute
111 Elm Street
Suite 103-105
Worcester, MA 01609
Ph: 508-755-3744
Fax: 508-770-0618
E-Mail: ayurveda@hotmail.com

International Federation of
Ayurveda — Dr. Krishna Kumar
27 Blight Street
Ridleyton S.A. 5008
Australia
Ph: 08-346-0631

Kaya Kalpa International
Dr. Raam Panday
111 Woodster Rd.
Satto, NY 10012

Life Impressions Institute
Attn: Donald VanHowten, Director
613 Kathryn Street
Santa Fe, NM 87501
Ph: 505-988-2627

Light Institute of Ayurveda
Dr's Bryan & Light Miller
P. O. Box 35284
Sarasota, FL 34242
E-Mail: earthess@aol.com
Web: ayurvedichealings.com

Lotus Ayurvedic Center
4145 Clares St. Suite D
Capitola, CA 95010
Ph: 408-479-1667

Maharishi Ayurved at the Raj
1734 Jasmine Avenue
Fairfield, IA 52556
Ph: 800-248-9050
Fax: 515-472-2496

Maharishi Health Center
Hale Clinic
7 Park Crescent
London, W14 3H3
England

Natural Therapeutics Center
Surya Daya
Gisingham, Nr. Iye
Suffolk, England

New England Institute of
Ayurvedic Medicine
111 N. Elm Street
Suites 103-105
Worcester, MA 01609
Ph: 508-755-3744
Fax: 508-770-0618
E-Mail: ayurveda@hotmail.com

Rocky Mountain Ayurveda
Health Retreat
P.O. Box 5192
Pagosa Springs, CO 81147
Ph: 800-247-9654 or 970-264-9224
E-Mail:
valentines@ayurveda-retreat.com
Web: www.ayurveda-retreat.com/
rockymountain

European Institute of Vedic Studies
Atreya Smith, Director
Ceven Point N° 230
4 bis rue Taisson
30100 Ales, France
Fax: 33-466-60-53-72
E-Mail: atreya@compuserve.com
Web: www.atreya.com

Victoria Stern, N.D.
P. O. Box 1814
Laguna Beach, CA 92652
Ph: 714-494-8858

Vinayak Ayurveda Center
2509 Virginia NE, Ste D
Albuquerque, NM 87110
Ph: 505-296-6522
Fax: 505-298-2932
Web: ayur.com

Wise Earth School of Ayurveda
Attn: Bri. Maya Tiwari
RR1 Box 484
Candler, NC 28715
Ph: 704-258-9999
Teachers and Practitioners Training
Programs Only.

Ayurvedic Cosmetic Companies

Auroma International
P. O. Box 1008
Dept. AM
Silver Lake, WI 53170
Ph: 262-889-8569
Fax: 262-889 8591
Importer and master distributor of Auroshikha Incense, Chandrika Ayurvedic Soap and Herbal Vedic Ayurvedic products.

Bindi Facial Skin Care
A Division of Pratima Inc.
109-17 72nd Road
Lower Level
Forest Hills, New York 11375
Ph: 718-268-7348

Devi Inc. (for Shivani product line)
Attn: Anjali Mahaldar
P. O. Box 377
Lancaster, MA 01523
Ph: 800-237-8221
Fax: 508-368-0455

Gajee Herbals
The Khenpo Company
Attn: Gayatri Puri, Owner
17595 Harvard St., C531
Irvine, CA 92714
Ph: 714-250-6027

Internatural
33719 116th St.
Box AM
Twin Lakes, WI 53181 USA
800-643 4221 (toll free order line)
262-889 8581 (office phone)
262-889 8591 (fax)
E-Mail:
internatural@lotuspress.com
Web: www.internatural.com
Retail mail order and internet reseller of essential oils, herbs, spices, supplements, herbal remedies, incense, books and other supplies.

Lotus Brands, Inc.
P. O. Box 325
Dept. AM
Twin Lakes, WI 53181
Ph: 262-889-8561
Fax: 262-889-8591
E-Mail:
lotusbrands@lotuspress.com
Manufacturer and distributor of natural personal care and herbal products, massage oils, essential oils, incense and aromatherapy items.

Lotus Light Enterprises
P. O. Box 1008
Dept. AM
Silver Lake, WI 53170 USA
800-548 3824 (toll free order line)
262-889 8501 (office phone)
262-889 8591 (fax)
E-Mail: lotuslight@lotuspress.com
Wholesale distributor of essential oils, herbs, spices, supplements, herbal remedies, incense, books and other supplies. Must supply resale certificate number or practitioner license to obtain catalog of more than 10,000 items.

Siddhi Ayurvedic Beauty Products
C/O Vinayak Ayurveda Center
2509 Virginia NE, Suite D
Albuquerque, NM 87110
Ph: 505-296-6522
Fax: 505-298-2932

Swami Sada Shiva Tirtha
Ayurvedic Holistic Center
82A Bayville Avenue
Bayville, NY 11709
Ph/Fax: 516-628-8200

TEJ Beauty Enterprises, Inc. (an Ayurvedic Beauty Salon)
162 West 56th St. Rm 201
New York, NY 10019
(owner: Pratima Raichur, founder of Bindi)
Ph: 212-581-8136

Ayurvedic Herbal Suppliers

Auroma International
P. O. Box 1008
Dept. AM
Silver Lake, WI 53170
Ph: 262-889-8569
fax: 262-889 8591
Importer and master distributor of Auroshikha Incense, Chandrika Ayurvedic Soap and Herbal Vedic Ayurvedic products.

Ayur Herbal Corporation
P. O. Box 6390
Santa Fe, NM 87502
Ph: 262-889-8569

Ayurveda Center of Santa Fe
1807 Second St., Suite 20
Santa Fe, NM 87505
Ph: 505-983-8898

Ayush Herbs, Inc.
10025 N.E. 4th Street
Bellevue, WA 98004
Ph: 800-925-1371

Banyan Trading Company
Traditional Ayurvedic Herbs - Wholesale
P. O. Box 13002
Albuquerque, NM 87192
Ph: 505-244-1880;
800-953-6424
Fax: 505-244-1878

Bazaar of India Imports, Inc.
1810 University Avenue
Berkeley, CA 94703
Ph: 800-261-7662; 510-548-4110

Dhanvantri Aushadhalaya
Herbs of Wisdom and Love,
Ayurvedic Herbs and Classical
Formulas.
P. O. Box 1654
San Anselmo, CA 94979
Ph: 415-289-7976
Email: ayurveda@dhanvantri.com

Dr. Singha's Mustard Bath and More
Attn: Anna Searles
Natural Therapeutic Centre
2500 Side Cove
Austin, TX 78704
Ph: 800-856-2862

Bio Veda
215 North Route 303
Congers, NY 10920-1726
Ph: 800-292-6002

Earth Essentials Florida
Dr's Bryan and Light Miller
4067 Shell Road
Sarasota, FL 34242
Ph: 941-316-0920

Frontier Herbs
P. O. Box 229
Norway, IA 52318
Ph: 800-669-3275

HerbalVedic Products
P. O. Box 6390
Santa Fe, NM 87502

Internatural
33719 116th St.
Box AM
Twin Lakes, WI 53181 USA
800-643-4221 (toll free order line)
262-889-8581 (office phone)
262-889-8591 (fax)
email: internatural@lotuspress.com
Web: www.internatural.com
Retail mail order and internet reseller of essential oils, herbs, spices, supplements, herbal remedies, incense, books and other supplies.

Kanak
P. O. Box 13653
Albuquerque, NM 87192-3653
Ph: 505-275-2469

Lotus Brands, Inc.
P. O. Box 325
Dept. AM
Twin Lakes, WI 53181

Ph: 262-889-8561
Fax: 262-889-8591

Lotus Herbs
1505 42nd Ave. Suite 19
Capitola, CA 95010
Ph: 408-479-1667

Lotus Light Enterprises
P. O. Box 1008
Dept. AM
Silver Lake, WI 53170 USA
800-548-3824 (toll free order line)
262-889-8501 (office phone)
262-889-8591 (fax)
email: lotuslight@lotuspress.com
Wholesale distributor of essential
oils, herbs, spices, supplements,
herbal remedies, incense, books
and other supplies. Must supply
resale certificate number or
practitioner license to obtain
catalog of more than 10,000 items.

Maharishi Ayurveda Products
International, Inc.
417 Bolton Road
P. O. Box 541
Lancaster, MA 01523
Info: 800-843-8332 Ext. 903
Order: 800-255-8332 Ext. 903

Planetary Formulations
P. O. Box 533
Soquel, CA 95073
Formulas by Dr. Michael Tierra.

Quantum Publication, Inc.
P. O. Box 1088
Sudbury, MA 01776
Ph: 800-858-1808

Seeds of Change
P. O. Box 15700
Santa Fe, NM 87506-5700
Catalog of rare Western and Indian
seeds.

Vinayak Panchakarma Chikitsalaya
Y.M.C.A Complex, Situbuldi
Nagpur (Maharastra State)
India 440 012

Ph: 011-91-712-538983
Fax: 011-91-712-552409
Retail/Wholesale

Yoga of Life Center
2726 Tramway N.E.
Albuquerque, NM 87122
Ph: 505-275-6141

The Center For Release
and Integration
450 Hillside Drive
Mill Valley, CA 94941

Dr. Jay Schererís Academy of
Natural Healing
1443 St. Francis Drive
Santa Fe, NM 87505

The Rolf Institute
205 Canyon Blvd.
Boulder, CO 80302

The Upledger Institute
1211 Prosperity Farms Rd.
Palm Beach Gardens, FL 33410

Correspondence Courses

Light Institute of Ayurveda
Teachers: Dr's Bryan & Light Miller
P. O. Box 35284
Sarasota, FL 34242
Ph: 941-346-3518
Fax: 941-346-0800
E-Mail: earthess@aol.com
Web: www.ayurvedichealing.com
Ayurvedic Pratitioner Training,
Correspondence Course, Books.

American Institute of Vedic Studies
Dr. David Frawley, Director
P. O. Box 8357
Santa Fe, NM 87504-8357
Ph: 505-983-9385
Fax: 505-982-5807
E-Mail: vedicinst@aol.com
Web: consciousnet.com/vedic
Correspondence courses in
Ayurveda and Vedic Astrology.

Lessons and Lectures in Ayurveda
by Dr. Robert Svoboda
P. O. Box 23445
Albuquerque, NM 87192-1445
Ph: 505-291-9698

Institute for Wholistic Education
33719 116th St.
Box AM
Twin Lakes, WI 53181
Ph: 262-877-9396

European Institute of Vedic Studies
Atreya Smith, Director
Ceven Point N° 230
4 bis rue Taisson
30100 Ales, France
Fax: 33-466-60-53-72
E-Mail: atreya@compuserve.com
Web: www.atreya.com
Represents David Frawley's courses
in Ayurveda in both French and
German languages.

To train in Ayurvedic Facial Massage and Beauty practices

Melanie Sachs — "Invoking Beauty
with Ayurveda" Seminars
P. O. Box 13753-3753
San Luis Obispo, CA 93406

Beauty and Quality Ayurvedic Supplements

Auroma International
P. O. Box 1008
Dept. AM
Silver Lake, WI 53170
Ph: 262-889-8569
fax: 262- 889 8591
Importer and master distributor of
Auroshikha Incense, Chandrika
Ayurvedic Soap and Herbal Vedic
Ayurvedic products.

Ayur Herbal Corporation
P. O. Box 6390 YA
Santa Fe, NM 87502

Ph: 262-889-8569
Fax: 262-889 8591
Manufacturer of Herbal Vedic
Ayurvedic products.

Internatural
33719 116th St.
Box AM
Twin Lakes, WI 53181 USA
800-643-4221 (toll free order line)
262-889-8581 (office phone)
262-889 8591 (fax)
E-Mail:
internatural@lotuspress.com
Web: www.internatural.com
Retail mail order and internet
reseller of essential oils, herbs,
spices, supplements, herbal
remedies, incense, books and other
supplies.

Lotus Brands, Inc.
P. O. Box 325
Dept. AM
Twin Lakes, WI 53181
Ph: 262-889-8561
Fax: 262-889-8591
E-Mail:
lotusbrands@lotuspress.com
Manufacturer and distributor of
natural personal care and herbal
products, massage oils, essential
oils, incense and aromatherapy
items.

Lotus Light Enterprises
P. O. Box 1008
Dept. AM
Silver Lake, WI 53170 USA
800-548-3824 (toll free order line)
262-889-8501 (office phone)
262-889-8591 (fax)
E-Mail: lotuslight@lotuspress.com
Wholesale distributor of essential
oils, herbs, spices, supplements,
herbal remedies, incense, books
and other supplies. Must supply
resale certificate number or
practitioner license to obtain
catalog of more than 10,000 items.

Maharishi Ayur-Veda Products
International, Inc.
417 Bolton Road
P. O. Box 54
Lancaster, MA 01523
Ph: 800-ALL-VEDA
Fax: 508-368-7475

New Moon Extracts
P. O. Box 1947
Brattleborough, VT 05302-1947
Ph: 800-543-7279

Spectrum Natural Omega 3 Oil
The Oil Company
133 Copeland Street
Petaluma, CA 94952

Universal Light, Inc.
P. O. Box 261
Dept. AM
Wilmot, WI 53192
Ph: 262-889 8571
Fax: 262-889 8591
Importer and Master Distributor
for Vicco Herbal Toothpaste.

Color, Sound, and Gems

PAZ
P. O. Box 4859
Albuquerque, NM 87196
For open-backed gemstone settings

Color Therapy Eyewear
C/O Terri Perrigone-Messer
P. O. Box 3114
Diamond Springs, CA 95619

Lumatron (light device)
C/O Ernie Baker
515 Pierce Street #3
San Francisco, CA 94117
Ph: 415-626-0083

Genesis (sound device)
Medical Massage Therapy
Attn: Tina Shinn
1857 Northwest Blvd. Annex
Columbus, Ohio 43212
Ph: 614-488-5244

Essential Oil Supplies

Aromatherapy Supply
Unit W3
The Knoll Business Center
Old Shoreham Road
Hove, Sussex BN3 7GS
England

Aroma Vera
3384 South Robertson Pl.
Los Angeles, CA 90034
Ph: 800-669-9514

Auroma International
P. O. Box 1008
Dept. AM
Silver Lake, WI 53170
Ph: 262-889-8569
fax: 262- 889 8591
Importer and master distributor of
Auroshikha Incense, Chandrika
Ayurvedic Soap and Herbal Vedic.

Ayurvedic Products

Earth Essentials Florida, Inc.
P. O. Box 35214
Sarasota, FL 34242
Ph: 800-370-3220
Fax: 941-346-0800
E-Mail: earthess@aol.com
Rare Essential Oils.

Fenmail Tisserand Oils
P. O. Box 48
Spalding, LINCS PE11 ADS
England

Internatural
33719 116th St.
Box AM
Twin Lakes, WI 53181 USA
800-643 4221 (toll free order line)
262-889 8581 (office phone)
262-889 8591 (fax)
E-Mail:
internatural@lotuspress.com
Web: www.internatural.com
Retail mail order and internet
reseller of essential oils, herbs,

spices, supplements, herbal remedies, incense, books and other supplies.

Lotus Brands, Inc.
P. O. Box 325
Dept. AM
Twin Lakes, WI 53181
Ph: 262-889-8561
Fax: 262-889-8591
E-Mail:
lotusbrands@lotuspress.com
Manufacturer and distributor of natural personal care and herbal products, massage oils, essential oils, incense and aromatherapy items.

Lotus Light Enterprises
P. O. Box 1008
Dept. AM
Silver Lake, WI 53170 USA
800-548 3824 (toll free order line)
262-889 8501 (office phone)
262-889 8591 (fax)
E-Mail: lotuslight@lotuspress.com
Wholesale distributor of essential oils, herbs, spices, supplements, herbal remedies, incense, books and other supplies. Must supply resale certificate number or practitioner license to obtain catalog of more than 10,000 items.

Private Universe
P. O. Box 3122
Winter Park, FL 32790
Ph: 407-644-7203

Oshadi Ayus - QualityLife Products
15, Monarch Bay Plaza, Suite 346
Monarch Beach, CA 92629
Ph: 800-947-1008
Fax: 714-240-1104

Primavera
D 8961 Sulzberg
Germany
08376-808-0

Original Swiss Aromatics
P. O. Box 606

San Rafael, CA 94915
Ph: 415-459-3998

Smitasha
26961 Ayamonte Dr.
Mission Viejo, CA 92692
Ph: 949-982-8777; 714-785-6891
Exercise Programs & Information.

Callanetic Headquarters
1700 Broadway
Suite 2000
Denver, CO 80290
Ph: 303-831-4455

Diamond Way Health Associates
214 Girard Blvd. NE
Albuquerque, NM 87106
Ph: 505-265-4826
(for Sotai, Tibetan Rejuvenation Exercises)

Partners Yoga
4876 Darvin Court
Boulder, CO 80301
Ph: 303-415-0199

Vega Study Center
1511 Robinson Street
Oroville, CA 95965
Ph: 916-533-7702
(for Sotai instructions - books)

Satori Resources
732 Hamlin Way
San Leandro, CA 94578
(for Tai Chi Chih)

Kushi Institute
P. O. Box 7
Becket, MA 01223
Ph: 413-623-5741
(for Do-in)

Natural Ingredients

Aloe Farms
P. O. Box 125
Los Fresnos, TX 78566
Ph: 800-262-6771
(for aloe vera juice, gel, powder and capsules)

Arya Laya Skin Care Center
Rolling Hills Estates, CA 90274
(for carrot oil)

Aubrey Organics
4419 North Manhattan Avenue
Tampa, FL 33614
(for rosa mosquita oil and a large
variety of natural cosmetics and
shampoos)

Body Shop
45 Horsehill Road
Cedar Knolls, NJ 07927-2014
Ph: 800-541-2535
(aloe vera, nut and seed oils,
cosmetics, make-up, brushes,
loofahs, and much more)

Culpepper Ltd.
21 Bruton Street
London W1X 7DA
England
(variety of natural seed, nut, and
kernal oils, essential oils, herbs,
books, and cosmetics)

Desert Whale Jojoba Co.
P. O. Box 41594
Tucson, AZ 85717
Ph: 602-882-4195
(for jojoba products and many
other natural oils, including rice
bran, pecan, macadamia nut and
apricot kernal)

Everybody Ltd.
1738 Pearl Street
Boulder, CO 80302
Ph: 800-748-5675
(large variety of oils, oil blends, and
cosmetics)

Flora Inc.
P. O. Box 950
805 East Badger Road
Lynden, WA 98264
Ph: 800-446-2110
(for flax seed oil, herbal supplements for skin, hair, nails and
cosmetics)

Green Earth Farm
P. O. Box 672
65 1/2 North 8th Street
Saguache, CO 81149
(for calendula oil, creme, and
herbal bath)

The Heritage Store, Inc.
P. O. Box 444
Virginia Beach, VA 23458
Ph: 804-428-0100
(castor oil, organic ghee, cocoa
butter, massage oils, flowerwaters,
essential oils, cosmetics, and
natural home remedies)

Internatural
33719 116th St.
Box AM
Twin Lakes, WI 53181 USA
800-643 4221 (toll free order line)
262-889 8581 (office phone)
262-889 8591 (fax)
E-Mail:
internatural@lotuspress.com
Web: www.internatural.com
Retail mail order and internet
reseller of essential oils, herbs,
spices, supplements, herbal
remedies, incense, books and other
supplies.

Janca's Jojoba Oil & Seed Company
456 E. Juanita #7
Mesa, AZ 85204
Ph: 602-497-9494
(jojoba oil, butter, wax, and seeds.
Also a large variety of naturally
pressed unusual oils, such as
camellia, kukui nut, and grapeseed.
Also have clay, aloe products,
essential oils, and their own line of
cosmetics)

Lotus Brands, Inc.
P. O. Box 325
Dept. AM
Twin Lakes, WI 53181
Ph: 262-889-8561
Fax: 262-889-8591
E-Mail:

lotusbrands@lotuspress.com
Manufacturer and distributor of natural personal care and herbal products, massage oils, essential oils, incense and aromatherapy items.

Lotus Light Enterprises
P. O. Box 1008
Dept. AM
Silver Lake, WI 53170 USA
800-548 3824 (toll free order line)
262-889 8501 (office ph.)
262-889 8591 (fax)
E-Mail: lotuslight@lotuspress.com
Wholesale distributor of essential oils, herbs, spices, supplements, herbal remedies, incense, books and other supplies. Must supply resale certificate number or practitioner license to obtain catalog of more than 10,000 items.

Weleda, Inc.
841 South Main Street
Spring Valley, NY 10977
(for calendula oil and a large variety of natural cosmetics)

Non-Denominational Meditation Training

Shambhala Training International
Executive Offices
1084 Tower Road
Halifax, Nova Scotia
Canada B3H 265

Organic Milk/Certified Raw Milk Suppliers

Alta Delta Certified Raw Milk
P. O. Box 388
City of Industry, CA 91747
Ph: 818-964-6401
(non pasteurized, non-homogenized milk)

Natural Horizons, Inc.
7490 Clubhouse Road

Boulder, CO 80301
Ph: 303-530-2711
(organic/pasteurized, non-homogenized milk; whole, low-fat, skim buttermilk and cream)

Organic Valley Family of Farms
C/O Cropp Cooperative
La Farge, WI
Ph: 608-625-2602
(organic butter, non-homogenized low-fat milk)

Pancha Karma Kitchen Equipment

Earth Fare
Attn: Roger Derrough
66 Westgate Parkway
Asheville, NC 28806
Ph: 704-253-7656
Carries hand grinders and suribachi clay pots and bowls.

Garber Hardware
49 Eighth Avenue
New York, NY 10014
Carries hand grinders, but no mail order.

Sesam Muhle Natural Products
RR1
Durham, Ontario
Canada, NOG 1RO
Ph: 519-369-6326
Carries a line of hand grinders and flakers for grains and legumes, made in Germany.

Taj Mahal Imports
1594 Woodcliff Drive, N.E.
Atlanta, GA 30329
Ph: 404-321-5940
Carries a full line of Indian kitchen equipment.

Pancha Karma Supplies

Vicki Stern
P. O. Box 1814
Laguna Beach, CA 92651

Ph: 714-494-8858
(for steam boxes)

To Receive Pancha Karma

Ayurvedic Healings
Dr's Bryan & Light Miller
P. O. Box 35284
Sarasota, FL 34242
Ph: 941-346-3518
Fax: 941-346-0800
E-Mail: earthess@aol.com
Web: www.ayurvedichealing.com
Panch Karma, Kaya Kalpa,
Jarpana, Shirodhara

Diamond Way Health Associates
214 Girard Blvd., NE
Albuquerque, NM 87106
Ph: 505-265-4826

Dr. Lobsang Rapgay
2931 Tilden Ave.
Los Angeles, CA 90064
Ph: 310-477-3877

Rocky Mountain Ayurveda
Health Retreat
P.O. Box 5192
Pagosa Springs, CO 81147
Ph: 800-247-9654 or 970-264-9224
E-Mail:
valentines@ayurveda-retreat.com
Web: www.ayurveda-retreat.com/
rockymountain

Spa Medicine

Ancient Way Ayurvedic Health Spa
Attn: Dr. Dennis Thompson
11510 N. Foothills HWY (Hwy 36)
Longmont, CO 80503
Ph: 303-823-0522; 800-601-9707
E-Mail: drtdrt@concentric.net

Transformational Seminars

ClearMind Institute
Duane O'Kane
22778 72nd Avenue
Langley, B.C., V2Y 2K3 Canada
Ph: 800-210-0372;
604-513-2219

Michael Rice
c/o Heartland
Rt. 3, Box 3280
Theodosia, MO 65761
Ph: 417-273-4838

Sandy Levey-Lunden
Skraddarod 24
272 97 Garsnas, Sweden
Phone: 011 46-414-24320
Fax: 011 46-414-24395
E-Mail: On.Purpose@Swipnet.se

Vedic Astrology

American Council of Vedic
Astrology (ACVA)
P. O. Box 2149
Sedona, AZ 86339
Ph: 800-900-6595; 520-282-6595
Fax: 520-282-6097
Web: vedicastrology.org
E-Mail: acva@sedona.net
Conferences, tutorial and training
programs.

American Institute of Vedic Studies
Dr. David Frawley, Director
P. O. Box 8357
Santa Fe, NM 87504-8357
Ph: 505-983-9385
Fax: 505-982-5807
E-Mail: vedicinst@aol.com
Web: consciousnet.com/vedic
Correspondence courses in
Ayurveda and Vedic Astrology.

Jeffrey Armstrong
4820 N. 35th St.
Phoenix, AZ 85018
Ph: 602-468-9448
Ayurvedic Astrologer, Author,
Lecturer, Teacher

Videos

Feldenkrais Resources
Ph: 800-765-1907

Wishing Well Video
P. O. Box 1008
Dept. AM
Silver Lake, WI 53170
Ph: 262-889-8501
(wholesale & retail)

Index